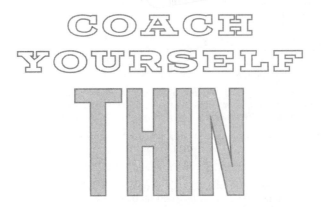

COACH YOURSELF THIN

FIVE STEPS TO RETRAIN YOUR MIND, RECLAIM YOUR POWER, AND LOSE THE WEIGHT FOR GOOD

GREG HOTTINGER, MPH, RD, and MICHAEL SCHOLTZ, MA

RODALE.

Notice

This book is intended as a reference volume only, not as a medical manual. The information given here is designed to help you make informed decisions about your health. It is not intended as a substitute for any treatment that may have been prescribed by your doctor. If you suspect that you have a medical problem, we urge you to seek competent medical help.

The information in this book is meant to supplement, not replace, proper exercise training. All forms of exercise pose some inherent risks. The editors and publisher advise readers to take full responsibility for their safety and know their limits. Before practicing the exercises in this book, be sure that your equipment is well-maintained, and do not take risks beyond your level of experience, aptitude, training, and fitness. The exercise and dietary programs in this book are not intended as a substitute for any exercise routine or dietary regimen that may have been prescribed by your doctor. As with all exercise and dietary programs, you should get your doctor's approval before beginning.

Mention of specific companies, organizations, or authorities in this book does not imply endorsement by the author or publisher, nor does mention of specific companies, organizations, or authorities imply that they endorse this book, its author, or the publisher.

Internet addresses and telephone numbers given in this book were accurate at the time it went to press.

© 2012 by Greg Hottinger and Michael Scholtz

All rights reserved. No part of this publication may be reproduced or transmitted in any form or by any means, electronic or mechanical, including photocopying, recording, or any other information storage and retrieval system, without the written permission of the publisher.

Rodale books may be purchased for business or promotional use or for special sales. For information, please write to: Special Markets Department, Rodale Inc., 733 Third Avenue, New York, NY 10017.

Printed in the United States of America

Rodale Inc. makes every effort to use acid-free ∞, recycled paper ♻.

Book design by Christina Gaugler

Library of Congress Cataloging-in-Publication Data

Hottinger, Greg.
    Coach yourself thin : five steps to retrain your mind, reclaim your power, and lose the weight for good / Greg Hottinger and Michael Scholtz.
        p.   cm.
    Includes bibliographical references and index.
    ISBN 978–1–60961–331–0   paperback
    1. Reducing diets—Popular works.   2. Weight loss—Popular works.   3. Nutrition—Psychological aspects—Popular works.   4. Physical fitness—Popular works. I. Scholtz, Michael. II. Title.
    RM222.2.H62   2011
    613.2'5—dc23   2011037756

Distributed to the trade by Macmillan

2   4   6   8   10   9   7   5   3   1   paperback

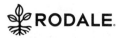

We inspire and enable people to improve their lives and the world around them.

www.rodalebooks.com

To Ali, Orijah, Jezai, and baby on the way.—Greg

To Tricia, Elizabeth, and Jason.—Michael

CONTENTS

INTRODUCTION

You may be wondering why you're even bothering with *another* weight-loss book. You've probably tried a number of the plans out there and are thinking skeptically to yourself, "What miracle are these guys offering up that's so different?"

We hear you loud and clear. We know you're frustrated with the promises in magazines, diet books, and on television; we know you're completely turned off by the guarantees made by exercise programs promising you a lean, hard body with no real work required. Finally, we understand that you're disappointed in yourself for not being able to lose weight and keep it off. But trust us when we say that the book you are holding in your hands is different. *Coach Yourself Thin* is not an extreme or fad diet, nor is it an intimidating, one-way-or-the-highway fitness plan. It is a guide that will help you identify the real-life obstacles that have been holding you back from losing weight; shift your thinking in ways that will remove those obstacles; and set personal goals that will lead to a healthy life—a life you may have given up hope of ever achieving.

We have worked with the overweight adult population for a combined 35 years, including 15 years at the Duke Diet & Fitness Center at Duke University. In 2001, we founded Novo Wellness (www.novowellness.com), a coaching and consulting practice; our goal at Novo is to help people achieve sustainable weight loss.

During our careers, we have seen failed weight-loss efforts more times than we can count. We've heard dieters complain of jumping from one plan to another—which usually ends up being just the same old diet and exercise rules in a new package—always with the hope of achieving better results. Though they may experience some level of success, it's usually short-term. Somehow, again and again, the pounds creep (or leap) back on.

When it comes to your own troubles with weight loss, you can probably cite a specific reason or a "triggering event" that has knocked you off track in the past. It may have been an illness or injury, or a vacation, move, or increased work stress. Faced with one of these, you fell off your diet and, with no recovery plan in place, you relapsed into old, unhealthy habits and patterns.

But what about individuals who are able to maintain healthy weights and healthy habits despite the curveballs life throws at them? Along with observing the more unfortunate weight-loss stories, we have also watched people get off the dieting roller coaster and move on to make beneficial changes to their lifestyles. Their victories make it clear that lasting weight loss is possible.

We argue that your overall *thinking,* not a specific triggering event, is the reason you haven't been able to lose weight and keep it off in the past. We have observed that our most successful clients use a similar set of behavioral skills and strategies that empower them to make consistently healthy choices. We want to share these important and powerful tools with you so you can shift your thinking and make your next weight-loss effort your last.

SETTING THE STAGE

In "Part 1: How Did It Come to This?" we take a look back at what has caused our current obesity epidemic and how most weight-loss plans perpetuate a way of thinking called the Quick Fix Mindset. This is precisely the kind of thinking that sabotages your efforts to lose weight. We also introduce the concept of coaching and discuss how the right balance of accountability and encouragement will help you overcome the obstacles that have held you back until now.

WHAT HAS STOPPED YOU IN YOUR TRACKS

In "Part 2: The Seven Undermining Obstacles to Weight Loss," you'll learn about the powerful thinking traps that lead people to give up on their diets, exercise plans, and themselves.

When your thinking patterns are "stuck," a triggering event can easily become your excuse to quit. But this time, you're going to be prepared. You're going to learn exactly which of the undermining obstacles are stopping you and then embark on a journey to overcome them.

LEARN HOW TO MOVE FORWARD

In "Part 3: The Five Stepping-Stones to Change," you'll learn the keys to overcoming any obstacle you face. Each of the five Stepping-Stones describes a powerful way of thinking that is crucial to your long-term success. While the paradigms are based on common sense, unlearning old mindsets and allowing yourself to experience these major shifts in your thinking takes some hard work.

To help you ease into changing the way you think, we have included "A-Ha" Exercises at the end of each Stepping-Stone. These are designed to help you get the feel of your new mindset and begin to experience the empowerment that comes with changing your perspective.

CHANGE YOUR RELATIONSHIP WITH FOOD AND EXERCISE

As you go through this process of change, you'll learn that it's not your diet plan that's the problem. The difference between failing and succeeding is in learning that it's actually your *relationship* with the plan that is getting in the way.

For this reason, in Part 4: Healthy Eating Guidelines, and Part 5: Healthy Exercise Guidelines, we introduce you to the basics of what it means to eat healthfully and to be active and fit. We outline the balanced approaches to eating and exercise that we believe to be the most effective and sustainable ways to reach your goals. These basics are all that you need to get on track and see dramatic changes in your health and weight—no crazy diet or gimmicks necessary.

In Part 4, you'll find a specific calorie structure and corresponding meal and snack suggestions that are based on your age, height, weight, and activity level. You are encouraged to use it to help you get on the right track as you develop the lifestyle eating pattern that will work for you in the years to come. Instead of a "one size fits all" routine, our Healthy Exercise Guidelines section describes what to look for in a good exercise plan and how to put together a plan that works for you. We introduce you to the fundamental components of exercise—daily activity, cardiovascular exercise, strength training, and rejuvenation.

CREATE LASTING CHANGE

Part 6 is called "Discovering Your Positive Inner Coach." Wellness coaching is a growing field of health care in which coaches help people reclaim control of their lives by empowering them to make their own choices.

We'll teach you how to be your own coach by using the same tools we use to help our own clients stay on track. The first section is "The Coach's Mental Toolbox," which is full of exercises and strategies for progressing through all five Stepping-Stones and driving home the powerful paradigm shifts contained in each. The second section, "Vision Building and Goal Setting," will show you how to create your own personal wellness vision—a vision of the life you want to lead. You will set goals to achieve that vision and learn how to adjust those goals to fit your unique circumstances, even as those circumstances evolve over time.

THE BEST WAY TO PROCEED

We've organized this book in the same way that you are most likely to change and grow: by first discovering the obstacles that hold you back, then learning how to overcome them, and finally applying your new, more empowered mindset for setting exciting future goals. However, don't feel obligated to read it straight through from beginning to end. If you want to set eating and exercise goals right from the start, feel free to turn to Parts 4 and 5 (see pages 115 and 183) and get rolling immediately. Think about some things that you'd like to change starting today, and if you need help, turn to "Vision Building and Goal Setting" (see page 250) for specific tips.

Whatever approach you take, *Coach Yourself Thin* will give you the knowledge and drive that you need to confront life's obstacles without letting them knock you off balance. You'll gain the tools and skills to begin coaching yourself through whatever life throws at you, and you'll finally get off the dieting roller coaster and lose the weight that has been holding you back. Eventually, your healthy lifestyle skills will be *unstoppable!*

Enjoy your journey,

Greg and Michael

PART 1

HOW DID IT COME TO THIS?

Just a few generations ago, Americans were not at all obsessed with weight. They didn't go on diets or have gym memberships, but they were actually leaner and stronger than most Americans are today. Their good health came naturally, in many respects, as their daily exercise was just part of their job at the railroad yard or factory. Similarly, healthy foods from the farm were often their only choices. As the years have passed, our job descriptions, the types of foods available to us, and our overall thinking have all shifted, pushing us further and further from the natural design that had helped stave off obesity for centuries. These shifts opened the door for a modern day health crisis.

CHAPTER 1

If Everyone Is Dieting, Why Are We Getting Fatter?

Ask your oldest living relatives about their life growing up and you might hear how exhausting it was to wake up with the roosters, go milk the cows, and bale hay all day long. You might hear about kids walking a couple of miles to and from school, actually *playing* during recess, and staying outside to play after school. In those days, you only stopped moving when your parents called you in for dinner. Most people who grew up in early 20th-century America were eating food fresh from the farm and getting plenty of daily activity. It was arguably the healthiest generation our country has ever seen.

Though it happened gradually, major changes have come our way over the course of the last 60 years. For most Americans, farm jobs, manual labor, and daily activity were replaced by office jobs, desk work, and

"One day, I overheard an overweight woman talking to her friend while walking up to the doors of their gym. 'Let's not do any more work than we have to,' she said as she pushed a button and stepped aside to make room for the automatic doors. I was struck by the irony of her comment—she was on her way to exercise but didn't want to exert the effort needed to open the doors." –Greg

labor-saving devices such as cars and dishwashers. These factors, especially the invention of the automobile, caused a significant decline in the amount of physical activity the average American experienced on a daily basis. And as our culture becomes more and more convenience-oriented, grocery delivery services and online shopping are making it easy to never leave home at all! What's more convenient than ordering a pizza from your couch and eating it in front of the movie you rented online?

MODERN DAY FOODS AND OUR VAST "WAIST LAND"

Equally detrimental to our health is the fact that while our energy expenditure has plummeted, the food processing industry has grown exponentially. During the late 20th century, the number of cheap, packaged products available in supermarkets exploded and the fast-food industry was born. Food became more accessible and plentiful than it had been at any other time in human history. And thanks to effective marketing on everything from billboards to radio to television, as well as the unrelenting use of the damaging food triple play—sugar, fat, and salt—we are now surrounded by products that are practically irresistible. Even if you are unusually strong-willed, it just takes one moment of weakness to find that you've inhaled a whopping 600 calories while driving or watching your favorite show.

Growing up in the '60s and '70s, we ate our share of sugary cereals, frozen TV dinners, canned soups, and other processed-food marvels. And like everyone else, we were so happy to have the convenience that we didn't question whether the ingredients in these foods might lead to serious health problems. It's remarkable that no one spoke up, when you consider that many of these foods were, and are still, made from refined flours, sugar, hydrogenated oils, and excessive amounts of salt, chemical fillers, and preservatives. The bottom line is that whether it snuck up on us or we simply chose to ignore this frightening trend, our families have been serving up meal after meal and snack after snack of these nutritionally empty foods for years.

Fake, Fattening Foods

There have been many health costs associated with America's widespread acceptance of processed foods. These include increased blood sugar and blood pressure levels, heart disease, and cancer.

But recent studies have revealed even bigger implications for the obesity epidemic. A person is much more likely to overeat when consuming a highly processed foods than when eating whole foods, especially if the fiber has been removed during the processing. This urge to overeat is not so much a conscious decision, but rather an autopilot physiological drive. Keeping a handful of potato chips from becoming the whole bag requires extraordinary self-control, and it doesn't help that everything has been supersized. Soft drinks, candy bars, fast-food meals, and even household staples like boxes of breakfast cereal have become enormous. Buying bigger usually means you get a better value, but it also means that you are likely to eat more. According to recent research, it's human nature to gobble down more candy from a huge package than a "fun-size" one. You are hard-wired to overeat when the opportunity is in front of you, and in our world, opportunity knocks often!

In a nutshell, processed foods are nearly impossible to eat in moderation, they're literally everywhere, and you can supersize them any time you like. Yikes! It's no wonder that society is fatter now than at any other time in history and that this change happened so quickly.

The implications of larger serving sizes, combined with our biological drive to overeat, are disastrous for a culture that faces large, extra-large, and jumbo-size portions throughout the day. Consider this: If you eat an extra 200 calories per day beyond what your body needs, at the end of a year you will have gained 20 pounds of fat. Many serving sizes have more than doubled in the last few decades. For example, in the 1970s, the standard fast-food order of a hamburger, fries, and a drink contained 650 calories, or about the same as today's regular hamburger, small fries, and small drink. However, if you supersize your order, your meal exceeds 1,400 calories!

But Wait, There's More

It's not hard to see how these changes translated into more people being overweight. It's all quite clear when you consider the "calories in versus calories out" equation: If you consume more calories than you expend, you gain weight. But the obesity epidemic is far more complex than simple math; in fact, it's shortsighted to include only food- and activity-related issues as the major contributors to the obesity problem. There is much more behind the obesity "perfect storm."

For example, increased stress and lack of sleep are both major players. And they are directly connected to one another: It's hard to sleep well when you are stressed-out, and you feel even more stressed when you're sleep deprived. It seems that everyone is battling intense job pressures in this ever-changing global economy, and some people are still struggling to make ends meet despite working more hours than ever. The human body is wired to go on full alert and kick into survival mode; this is commonly referred to as the fight-or-flight response. One hundred years ago, most jobs were physically demanding and provided a healthy outlet for stress, but today there are few natural outlets. If you're not making it to the gym regularly, the stress simply builds up, and chronic elevation of stress hormones has been implicated as a major factor in weight gain. High levels of stress lead to stress eating, a type of emotional eating that can wreak havoc with your food choices and your ability to discern real physical hunger from psychological hunger.

And on top of all that, chronic stress carries over into the night, interfering with both the quantity and quality of your sleep. This is bad news because studies have shown that people who get 7 to 9 hours of quality sleep each night are thinner than those who get fewer than 7 hours.

All of these factors have turned the health of modern day America into a vast "Waist Land." And while many questions remain about how to change the larger cultural picture, one thing appears certain: Simply going along with the ultraconvenient, supersedentary way of life is the fastest way to "supersize" yourself.

CHAPTER 2

The Quick Fix Mindset

Your whole life you have been told by advertisers that you can and should buy whatever you want, whenever you want it. You are sold on the idea that you deserve to indulge yourself and that having better, newer, and more stuff will "improve" the quality of your life. Not coincidentally, during the latter half of the twentieth century, there was an explosion in the availability of consumer goods and services. Even in most small towns, you can find a store with exactly what you're looking for, at almost any hour of the day; now with Internet shopping, you have even more options. To help facilitate your purchasing power, you have been extended credit to buy things, even if you can't afford them. There is no reason at all to wait if there is something you want right now. This is the heart of what we call the Quick Fix Mindset: the simple belief that anything can be yours with little effort and no consequence, and that you deserve to have it right now.

During the same time period described above, we had increased access to labor-saving tools and ideas and convenient, prepackaged meals: for example, "improvements" such as a riding lawn mower and the fast-food drive-thru window. With this increased desire for ease and convenience, the Quick Fix Mindset began adversely affecting people's choices and decisions about their health. The desire for more and more convenience took away our opportunities, and eventually our desire, to move and to nourish ourselves with healthy foods. These changes have undeniably accelerated the current health crisis.

However, the most destructive aspect of the Quick Fix Mindset—and the one that makes it a major obstacle to lifestyle change—is that the things touted as solutions are actually quick fixes themselves. In fact, it may feel as if you are stuck on a pendulum of Quick Fix thinking. At one extreme you overindulge in food and inactivity, using this as a way to cope with the pressures of modern life. At the other extreme are behaviors intended to counterbalance these indulgences—a result of the rush of panic that hits you when you wake up to how horrible you feel, how out of shape you've become, or how big you've gotten. You become determined to "fix" it—and fast—through rigid, restrictive diets and intense exercise regimens. And this approach, of course, backfires. And back you swing toward abuse and indulgence. Unless you transform your Quick Fix Mindset, you'll desperately swing from one extreme to the other with no end in sight.

EXAMPLES OF QUICK FIX THINKING

The following behaviors are some of the ways Quick Fix Thinking can manifest itself in your life.

- Taking medications at the least sign of discomfort or resorting to diet pills or invasive weight-loss surgery without making any lifestyle changes.
- Diving blindly into crazy exercise programs only to injure yourself and have to return to your sedentary lifestyle.
- Looking for every imaginable shortcut in daily tasks but spending hundreds of dollars on gym memberships and exercise equipment.
- Buying prepackaged foods instead of taking the time and effort to cook meals that include whole foods.

Quick Fix Thinking distracts you from doing the hard work of changing the unhealthy behaviors that are the root cause of weight gain. Instead, you continue to look to the "experts" to come up with a way to make the process simpler. And, of course, they oblige by continuing to try to sell you on the idea that weight loss should be quick and require minimal effort. Unfortunately, as you will see in Chapter 3, their answers haven't led to any real and lasting solutions.

"Experts" Who Don't Have the Answers

Though all of the so-called diet and weight-loss "secrets" flying around today fail to offer anything that is either new or helpful, the so-called experts continue to blast away with a barrage of new breakthroughs. Typically, diets and exercise methods that become big hits will pitch the idea that you can achieve your goal weight without changing much at all, use "smoke and mirrors" to sell a breakthrough where none exists, or do a little of both. We recently saw an ad for a diet program that promised you could lose weight and eliminate food cravings effortlessly, without counting calories or restricting the foods you eat.

Some plans have legitimate science behind them and yet seem unwilling to stick to the whole truth. This smoke-and-mirrors mentality refers to any diet and exercise idea that takes a little bit of truth and tries to turn it into groundbreaking news for weight loss. High-protein diets, for example, blame carbohydrates for the weight-gain epidemic and encourage dieters to eliminate carbs completely rather than just focus on reducing the amount of refined carbohydrates. This is smoke and mirrors because while drastically reducing carb intake can produce impressive weight loss, the results are only short-term because giving up most whole grains, dairy products, and fruits from the diet isn't sustainable for the majority.

Another example of a smoke-and-mirrors breakthrough came on the heels of research that showed your body selectively burns more fat when you exercise on an empty stomach. Many "experts" took that a step too far, claiming that exercising on an empty stomach is the best fat-burning method ever discovered. The problem with that claim is you can't burn more fat if you run out of gas. If you are pushing yourself with nothing in the tank, instead of burning more fat, you are likely to feel dizzy and weak from low blood sugar, which will stop your workout *and* calorie-burning in its tracks. Rather than look for a "loophole" to trick the body, follow the lead of the leanest and most fit athletes in the world who eat healthfully to fuel challenging and effective workouts.

And some weight loss programs combine the no-effort-required and smoke-and-mirrors techniques. For example, whole body vibration machines are touted as a way to easily build your core muscles. The claim is that you can build muscle and boost your metabolism by following a "gentle program that can be accomplished in as little as 10 minutes per day, 3 days per week." While it is true that these machines can challenge your muscles in very demanding ways and improve the strength of your core muscles, including your abdomen, lower back, and hips, you'll need to work harder than "gently" for 30 minutes per week if you want to look like the professional athletes featured in the ads. The smoke-and-mirrors aspect capitalizes on the fact that muscle mass is important to maintaining a strong metabolism. But the truth is you are not going to gain muscle mass while you lose weight, especially not in your core muscles, as many of the ads claim.

The Genetic or Hormonal Influence

There are a number of genetic and hormonal factors that explain why some people gain weight more readily and have a harder time losing it than others do, and these factors also explain why the same diet and exercise approach won't work the same way for everyone. But if genetics or hormonal imbalances were the biggest keys to the obesity epidemic, then there should have been the same percentage of overweight or obese people 100 years ago. As Dr. Elliot Joslin, founder of the Joslin Diabetes Center, puts it: "Genes load the gun. Lifestyle pulls the trigger."

THE "DIETS DON'T WORK" CAMP

As we've discussed, many people and so-called experts believe that a healthy weight can be achieved through a miracle or breakthrough diet. On the opposite end of the spectrum, however, are those who believe that to achieve weight loss, we must put an end to dieting altogether. This "no-diet" idea spread among people who were fed up with one diet after another failing to produce lasting results, and it really took the spotlight as weight-loss experts and nutritionists began to speak out about the dangers of severe calorie restriction and eliminating necessary food groups.

Thus was born what we call the Diets Don't Work movement, which holds the view that every attempt to diet will be fruitless: Diets have been around forever, everybody seems to be on one, and yet nobody appears to be losing and keeping off their weight.

The good news is that the Diets Don't Work movement has helped people move away from unsustainable diets. The bad news is that what the Diets Don't Work approach has to offer in terms of weight loss has been a colossal failure. Why? Because once you look behind the curtain, the only "new" idea in the Diets Don't Work arsenal is healthy eating in moderation and more exercise, which isn't structured enough to keep most people's attention. The pressure to eat unhealthy foods is too great, and the temptation is too ingrained for the simple guideline of eating in moderation to take hold. It works great, right up to the point where you don't want to do it anymore. After this, you're back to square one, wondering what's next. The solution comes down to making changes to the way you *think* rather than just finding a new way to diet. And this is where we can help you. What you'll discover is that the real solution is to find a balanced and healthy way to eat and exercise and then do the mental work necessary to continue these behaviors for the rest of your life. That is what *Coach Yourself Thin* is all about: showing you how to consistently do what is truly healthy. And it will change your life for good.

THE *COACH YOURSELF THIN* CHALLENGE

Losing weight and maintaining a healthy body weight is as easy as mastering the "eat-less, move-more" mantra and as tough as overcoming the obstacles and habits that perpetuate the "eat-more, move-less" reality we live in today.

To achieve lasting change and stay focused on what works, embrace these three tenets.

1. There are no holy grail diets or easy solutions. There is no perfect combination of foods that will magically take you to your ideal weight forever.

2. Weight loss comes down to eating healthy foods in appropriate amounts and being active on a regular basis.

3. Only by assessing your lifestyle and finding a healthy, balanced eating plan and livable approach to exercise can you find a plan that you will stick to.

It's hard work, but the payoffs are big. If you're ready for the challenge, read on.

CHAPTER 4

Seeing the Light— The Coach Approach

Once you are able to stop buying into the exaggerations and smoke and mirrors pitches and focus on the three tenets of what really works (see page 12), you'll still need two things to be successful. First, you'll need a healthy, balanced, and sustainable eating and exercise plan. We provide the tools you need to design these in Parts 4 and 5. Second, and even more importantly, you'll need to be consistent with your healthy behaviors.

The key to consistency, we believe, is looking inward. *You* are the expert. The moment that you stop looking "out there" for answers, you'll become noticeably more powerful, and self-empowerment leads to determination, motivation, confidence, persistence, and—ultimately—full control of your life and your decisions.

How do you make this transformation? In a word: coaching.

WHY YOU NEED COACHING

Coaching is the most powerful concept we have ever encountered in the field of lifestyle change. It is based on the idea that the answers you need to live a healthy life are found within you, not externally. Sure, a doctor can give you vital information and advice, but a coach will consider all of your strengths and weaknesses, your personal likes and dislikes, and your readiness to make changes, and he or she will use all of this information to help you unleash your full potential.

If you are interested in hiring a wellness coach and have the financial resources to do so, see page 273 for our recommendations on where to choose one. Having someone to bounce ideas off of and to help you facilitate change is invaluable. Our goal with this book is not to replace the role of a wellness coach, but to help you develop your own internal coaching voice. This is the single most important weapon you can have in your weight-loss arsenal.

Moving forward, *you* will be responsible for choosing what works for you. You'll no longer have to follow someone else's rules. You'll never have to eliminate foods like carrots, cake, bread, or pizza just because they are on someone else's no-no list! Instead of your old dieting mentality, you'll learn a whole new approach to change. The Coach Yourself Thin approach offers a refreshing alternative to an outdated and ineffective way of thinking. Here are a few examples.

- **Diet thinking** tells you that some foods should be avoided at all costs.
  The Coach Approach is that there are no good or bad foods. You'll learn to say yes to yourself without guilt, and what you want to say yes to will become healthier as you leave the guilt behind.

- **Diet thinking** tells you that you can quit your plan today and start over tomorrow.
  The Coach Approach is not a set-in-stone program to follow or to fall off. A lifestyle evolves from one day to the next, and you can make adjustments as needed, taking into account your victories and your setbacks.

- **Diet thinking** makes you believe that you have to be hard on yourself to change and that negative emotions like disgust and anger are motivators.
  The Coach Approach is that negative thoughts don't lead to change. Transformation is the result of positive feelings that build you up rather than tear you down, so improving your self-esteem and confidence actually precedes weight-loss success.

- **Diet thinking** says that diving in with both feet and pushing yourself to the max both lead to greater success.
  The Coach Approach is that you may need to lower the bar in order to jump over it. Keeping your weight-loss expectations realistic from the get-go will motivate you to move forward instead of frustrating you so much that you give up before you've even

started. You can continue to increase your standards as you make progress and gain confidence in your abilities.

Begin your journey to a slimmer, stronger, and healthier you by taking the pledge below.

Coach Yourself Thin *Pledge*

I have the power to change my relationship with food and exercise and my beliefs about myself, and I choose to begin living a healthier life starting today. I will let go of past failures and frustrations and instead focus on the choices and behaviors that I can control.

I believe that I can reach my health and weight-loss goals, and I will not be stopped by slow weight loss, a plateau, or the actions or opinions of those who do not support the changes I am making.

I know that changing is a journey that takes time, and I am willing to put in the necessary effort and be patient with myself. I believe in the path that I am on.

_____

SIGNATURE

_____

DATE

PART 2

THE SEVEN UNDERMINING OBSTACLES TO WEIGHT LOSS

During one or more of your previous efforts to lose weight, you may have experienced a sort of nirvana: a golden age where everything felt easy and having a positive outlook and being in control seemed to come naturally. Then, suddenly, the whole thing fell apart and you were left searching for what caused the crash.

In our experience, the majority of dieters locate and ultimately blame a triggering event for knocking them off track, mistakenly believing, as you might, that all would have gone just fine if not for this occurrence.

In our experience, it is not one event that knocks people off track. Over and over we see this theory rejected by people who succeed in the face of a major event or several simultaneous or consecutive events. Instead, we believe that your thinking is what holds you back. We have categorized the primary stumbling blocks—the Undermining Obstacles to Weight Loss—that sabotage you and keep you from having lasting success. As you read Part 2 of this book, you will explore these obstacles and the ineffective ways of thinking within each. Take time to read about each obstacle carefully: This is your chance to gain an understanding of your unique barriers to success and to begin mapping your pathway to truly sustainable weight loss.

Each chapter in this part starts with a short definition of the obstacle and an undermining thought that helps illustrate one aspect of the "stuck" thinking typical of the obstacle. We include a short quiz to help you determine if the obstacle in question is powerful in your life. In the quizzes, answer yes or no to each statement to indicate whether or not it applies to you. The more yes answers you have, the more likely it is that the obstacle in question is an important one to you. You can keep tabs on any changes by revisiting the quizzes periodically. In Part 3 we will explore the Five Stepping-Stones to Change and you will begin to develop new, more powerful and effective ways of thinking to help you overcome these obstacles.

CHAPTER 5

Weight Fixation

Definition: Being so focused on the number that pops up when you step on the scale that it interferes with your ability to stay consistent with your program and see the progress that you may in fact be making.

Undermining Thought: "If the number on the scale doesn't move, all of my efforts this week were for nothing."

Weight Fixation Quiz

1. I weigh myself more than once a day. Yes/No
2. I do not feel that I am succeeding unless the number on the scale drops, even if I have experienced other noticeable improvements (such as increased energy, reduced anxiety, improved endurance, or better sleep and digestion). Yes/No
3. I get upset if I weigh myself on a different scale—at my doctor's office, at the gym—and it shows that I'm heavier than on my scale at home. Yes/No
4. When my weight loss plateaus, I question whether or not I should continue with the program or quit altogether. Yes/No
5. I am not satisfied with losing only 1 to 2 pounds per week. Yes/No
6. I want to know the exact number of calories I burn during a workout. Yes/No
7. I often exercise until I "burn off" the calories I've eaten. Yes/No
8. If I miss a day of exercise, I do more exercise the next day to make up for it. Yes/No

9. I will choose a lower-calorie food even if the lower-calorie choice is more processed and not as healthy. Yes/No

10. I believe I will be totally happy once I reach my goal weight. Yes/No

Note: The *Coach Yourself Thin* quizzes are not to be used for diagnostic purposes. They are meant solely to give you information about the psychological and/or behavioral obstacles that may be holding you back from reaching your weight-loss goals.

THE NEED FOR SPEED

In a weight-loss environment dominated by the Quick Fix Mindset, where each diet and exercise program sells itself on the promise of being able to help you lose weight faster than the next plan, it's no wonder you're so focused on the scale or jeans sizes.

You can achieve fast weight loss through severe calorie restriction, excessive exercise, or diet pills, but such measures put a tremendous amount of unhealthy stress on your body, and the results *do not* last. You will not only gain back the weight you lost, you'll probably even add on a couple of extra pounds. A starved or overworked body doesn't understand that it's been put on a temporary diet. It interprets your actions as a threat and responds by slowing down your metabolism, releasing stress hormones, and, eventually, leading you to a food binge, an injury, or burnout—any of which can derail your diet for good.

LOOKING GOOD!

Weight Fixation is also driven by the fact that it feels good to be noticed. Apparently the immortal words of Billy Crystal's Fernando character on *Saturday Night Live* still ring true for many people: "It is better to look good than to feel good." Sadly, most people you run into won't point out your improved energy, stellar fitness, or happier mood—they'll compliment your shrinking waistline. And when you stop getting those compliments, your ambition goes right out the window. As one of our clients put it, "I just lost my motivation once people stopped commenting on how much weight I'd lost and how good I looked."

Will Weighing Less Often "Cure" Weight Fixation?

Not necessarily. For some, going longer between weigh-ins actually increases the desire and the pressure to lose even more weight from one weigh-in to the next. Daily weighing can work well if you are able to see your weight as just one piece of feedback among many, including your mood, energy level, confidence, physical strength, and endurance. If you have this mindset, the scale becomes just another tool, instead of judge and jury. In the end, that is the solution to Weight Fixation.

THE SCALE IS A DICTATOR

If you struggle with Weight Fixation, you might experience turbulent mood swings and engage in erratic, unhealthy behaviors that can set you up for falling off the wagon. Maybe you have a gigantic dessert the night before you begin your diet or you radically slash calories the day or two before your weigh-in. Maybe you are crushed because you've worked so hard for days and the scale hasn't budged, even though you step on it several times a day. The scale has so much power over you that it can delight you one moment, devastate you the next, and fill you with dread the morning of your weigh-in day.

Weight Fixation attaches your self-esteem and your motivation to the number on the scale. Ultimately, this means that if you are losing weight on "schedule," you'll continue with your program. Otherwise, you'll bail out before your program can even get off the ground and write it off as another failed diet attempt.

CHAPTER 6

All-or-Nothing Thinking

Definition: Believing that you need to follow your diet and exercise plan perfectly to successfully lose weight.

Undermining Thought: "If I don't push myself to the max and follow the rules to the letter—measure all my portions, write down everything I eat, exercise every time I should—then I won't lose weight!"

All-or-Nothing Thinking Quiz

1. I constantly "start over" with my diet and exercise plan. Yes/No

2. I typically want to speed up the weight-loss process, and I'm proud when I eat less or exercise more than my plan suggests. Yes/No

3. I expect to suffer and feel deprived in order to reach my weight-loss goal. Yes/No

4. I like the idea of eliminating certain foods or entire food groups to achieve faster weight loss. Yes/No

5. Deviating from my plan makes me feel like I've blown it and often results in my quitting. Yes/No

6. I rationalize unhealthy behaviors, such as having an extra dessert, a double portion, or being too busy to exercise by telling myself that I will make up for it by skipping meals or doubling up on my exercise later. Yes/No

7. I use the words "good" and "bad" to describe certain foods, my eating behaviors, and myself ("I was bad today, I ate cake"). Yes/No

8. I struggle with feelings of guilt, always thinking that I could be doing better. Yes/No

9. I believe in the mantra, "No pain, no gain." Yes/No

10. I like to begin a new program on a Monday. Yes/No

WE LOVE IT WHEN IT SPARKLES

It's a natural human instinct to be very excited about things that are brand new. Think about the last car you bought. You probably worked hard to keep your new ride sparkling—washing and waxing it constantly and laying down the law with the kids: "No food in that back seat!" Maybe you even invested in some new-car-smell spray to keep the feeling alive.

But that brand-newness doesn't last. First the car gets a scratch, then it needs new brakes, and eventually—no matter how hard you polish it—it doesn't shine the way that it did when you first brought it home. Eventually, your enthusiasm wears off. Then you forget to wash it on Saturday, and on Monday you look around in disbelief, wondering how all those chip bags and slushie cups ended up on the floor.

I'LL DO WHATEVER IT TAKES

People starting a new diet are like new-car owners: Being diligent about maintenance is exciting in the beginning! There is plenty of motivation to follow the plan exactly and stick with it no matter what. The newness makes the work involved feel easier, and enthusiasm and momentum cover up the amount of effort that you're putting in.

This zeal, combined with the Quick Fix Mindset, creates a heady potion, and it can be nearly impossible to resist the pull of All-or-Nothing Thinking. You are drawn to punishing exercise plans, you strive for perfection in your eating habits, and you cannot see any problem with going overboard because it all feels so good. For a while, you might even think that your plan is easy.

NOT SO FAST!

Soon, though, you're faced with challenges and you realize that you can't keep up the pace. Maybe you suddenly can't stand the fact that you're supposed to eat fish four times a week, or maybe you're on a diet that has no eating-out options and you find yourself with no time to cook, or you've started a running program only to discover that you hate running. You begin to battle thoughts such as, "I'm getting tired of these same old foods that I have to eat," and "I'd give anything for a bag of chips." Your fitness routine gets a bit tedious, and the muscle soreness that felt good before now just aches. Then work gets hectic, the laundry piles up, and it suddenly feels like you just can't handle this diet on top of all the other demands in your life. That's when you realize that things have gotten way out of control.

The more gung ho and extreme your initial effort, the greater the chance that you will swing to the other extreme as soon as you hit a rough patch. You go from eating wild salmon, quinoa, and kale to downing cheeseburgers, fries, and regular sodas, or from exercising like mad to being mad that you have to exercise.

CHAPTER 7

Feelings of Unworthiness

Definition: Negative, damaging beliefs about yourself or your body that undermine your self-esteem and make you believe that your diet, exercise, and weight-loss goals are unattainable or unimportant, or that you're not worthy of achieving them.

Undermining Thought: "I hate my thighs. They're disgusting to me. I'd give anything to have pretty legs."

Feelings of Unworthiness Quiz

1. My plans to exercise or eat a healthy meal often get interrupted by more important plans. Yes/No

2. I take care of family members and friends to the point that I don't have much time for myself. Yes/No

3. I feel guilty when I do something for myself. Yes/No

4. I feel best about myself when I am helping others. Yes/No

5. I feel unworthy of praise, attention, or success. Yes/No

6. Losing weight frightens me. Yes/No

7. I know it's just a matter of time until I "fall off the wagon." Yes/No

8. I don't like spending extra money on foods that are supposed to be healthier. Yes/No

9. I feel a bit safer around the opposite sex when I am on the heavier side. Yes/No

10. I believe it's selfish and a waste of money to pamper myself with things like massages, manicures, personal training, and yoga classes. Yes/No

NEGATIVITY EVERYWHERE YOU TURN

Unfortunately, negative feelings about your looks, weight, and body shape are fed by the same destructive advertising machine that spawned the Quick Fix Mindset. Slick marketing has sold our society the idea that if you are skinny and beautiful you will be considered socially acceptable, attractive, and a better candidate for a happy, successful life. This is now a common, deep-seated cultural belief for many people. If you are over-weight, you likely struggle with these harmful biases every day and may be faced with prejudice from others.

The real damage, however, is self-induced. The hurtful weapons wielded against you by someone else become massively destructive when you turn them against yourself. When this happens, you are disgusted by how you look and you end up missing out on some moments—such as hav-ing your picture taken with friends and family—that you would cherish forever. Or if you call yourself "fatty" or something worse in an effort to motivate yourself to go to the gym, it backfires, leaving you angry, resent-ful, and back on the couch.

THE FUTILITY OF YOUR DREAM WEIGHT

If you are like many of our clients, you may be longing for a body weight or shape that you have not seen for years—if ever. Perhaps you can't let go of a particular number on the scale, or maybe you have a certain clothing size that defines "skinny" to you. Maybe you see a movie star and set his or her "look" as your goal. Whatever the motive, you know that if you can just get there you will look good, be desirable, and finally win acceptance.

However, if you think back on a time when you may have hit that magical number or size in the past, you probably weren't truly happy then, either. You probably still wished you weighed something less or had plans to drop another size. Weight loss is relative; often the only thing that is consistent is the desire to lose more. The sad thing is being unhappy with yourself at your current weight will only lead to more weight gain down the road. And if you reach some higher number, you will probably long for the weight you are today.

It is crazy how your perception changes, isn't it? You can be unhappy with a particular weight as you pass it on your way to being heavier, and later you feel like that same weight would make you happy, if you could just get there again.

The truth is that when your image of yourself is tied to your weight and you feel disgusted and frustrated by that weight, the number on the scale matters little. Until you make peace with your body, you will always want to lose more and be paralyzed by the fear of getting heavier.

PUTTING LIFE ON HOLD

When you experience Feelings of Unworthiness, you are in a sense postponing your life, believing that it will get much better when you get to your goal weight. But until then, you don't feel that you should enjoy yourself or that you deserve to be happy. You stay away from social situations whenever you can, you hold back from fun physical activities, and you put off starting new relationships. You are certain nobody would want to go out with you at your current weight. Feelings of Unworthiness can even *cause* you to gain weight in an effort to feel safer and more "protected" from the opposite sex. Extra body weight can act as a shield to deflect potential suitors or can be used as an excuse for the lack of intimacy.

Your self-doubt even keeps you from taking care of your health. Since you go out of your way to avoid exposing yourself to others' criticism, you refuse to exercise in a group class or gym, or even to take a walk in your neighborhood, and you wouldn't be caught dead swimming laps at the pool.

PUTTING YOUR NEEDS LAST

Feelings of Unworthiness may lead you to place the needs of others before your own. Maybe you're a great cook, an excellent parent, or a dutiful caretaker. You focus on the areas of your life where you feel more confident, competent, and needed so you can deflect attention from your weight and give yourself an excuse not to work on it. You're unable to take any action to change your health in a meaningful and lasting way because it's easier and more rewarding to seek out the situations where you feel good about yourself than it is to try to change an area where you don't.

RELYING ON "TOUGH LOVE"

Feelings of Unworthiness can cause you to take a tough love approach to losing weight. Maybe you think, "I have to be hard on myself, or I will just eat the whole world," or "I'd never move if I didn't force myself." It's as if you're disciplining an unruly child who'll sneak off and do something wrong if you don't constantly watch her.

The problem is that, as with an unruly child, the harder you push yourself, the more likely you are to push back. You can force yourself to exercise for a while, but eventually you'll begin finding ways to get out of it. Maybe you'll do too much and get hurt. Or you might "forget." Or perhaps you'll schedule something "more important" during your exercise time.

> "There is a constant stream of 'I want food!' running through my head. I need to change that stream of chatter in my head and replace it with something different like, 'You just ate!' or 'You aren't hungry!' or 'You don't need food right now!' or 'Dinner (or my next meal or snack) is only 2 hours away, you're not going to pass out before then.'"
>
> —*Biggest Loser Club member*

You will also find that tough love offers little comfort and no boost to confidence in situations where what you really need is empathy and understanding. For example, at first glance, it may seem like the example above is a good way to replace a craving with thoughts to help counteract it. But, from a coach's perspective, this self-talk is not positive at all: It's very negative, condescending, and demanding. It's like telling a child who comes to you scared to death of the dark, "It's not so dark, you're not scared, and daybreak is coming soon." This approach offers no help in overcoming the root of the problem, whether it is a craving *or* a fear of the dark.

Tough love offers little comfort and no boost to confidence in a situation like this!

CHAPTER 8

Resisting Responsibility

Definition: Blaming external circumstances for why you are unable to make healthy lifestyle choices.

Undermining Thought: "I can't stay on any diet because my co-workers keep bringing doughnuts to the office."

Resisting Responsibility Quiz

1. I believe that some people can eat whatever they want and not exercise and still be healthy. Yes/No

2. I can't lose weight no matter how hard I try. Yes/No

3. I find myself waiting for the "right time" to begin eating healthy and exercising. Yes/No

4. I wish I didn't, but I prefer junk food to healthy food. Yes/No

5. It gets way too hot/cold here in the summer/winter. There's no way I can exercise in the heat/cold. Yes/No

6. I wish I could quit my job and just focus on me. Yes/No

7. If I had a good trainer, I know I could lose weight. Yes/No

8. I am jealous of people who seem to truly enjoy exercise. Yes/No

9. When I lost my workout partner, I got out of the habit of exercising. Yes/No

10. When my friends want to eat at restaurants with burgers and fries and not a salad in sight, I always end up going along and making bad food choices. Yes/No

WHAT'S YOUR EXCUSE?

The Quick Fix Mindset leads you to believe that weight loss is supposed to be easy. The media shows you image after image of beautiful people who, by all appearances, have been wildly successful with their diet and exercise programs.

You begin thinking that there must be something wrong with you for not achieving those same results, so you look for explanations. You blame your thyroid, your metabolism, or your genes. Or you make excuses for why you can't stick with your plan: It's too hot or too cold out, you're too busy, or your food choices are too bland or too expensive. In the end, feeling frustrated by not being able to lose weight as easily as you think you should keeps you from consistently practicing the healthy behaviors that *do* lead to weight loss.

WHO'S IN CHARGE?

Resisting Responsibility for your choices opens the door for other people— particularly those with whom you share a home or office—to take control of the decisions you make about food and exercise. When those around you do not share your commitment to a healthy lifestyle, the most basic actions, such as buying groceries, cooking meals, going out to eat, and finding time to exercise, can become points of contention. It also gives you the opportunity to use them as an excuse as to why you aren't making better choices.

All of these situations can be stressful, and you may feel pressure to give up your healthy choices or feel that they are too much trouble to stick with. But ultimately, the decisions you make are up to you. It is only by giving up your right to stand up for your needs, ask for help, and seek support that you allow those decisions to be governed by someone else.

To eat healthfully, you may need to buy separate groceries or cook separately. Or, if you go to the restaurants that your friends or family prefer, you may need to skip certain foods or sit patiently and watch them eat and drink while you wait to go home and eat healthier foods. And if those around you don't exercise, you may feel like you have to excuse yourself from what everyone else is doing while you go exercise.

NOWHERE TO TURN

Resisting Responsibility also means that you allow your physical environment and personal circumstances to hinder healthy decision-making. You may believe that you live in an area with too much pollution and too little green space for you to exercise outside or your gym is too far away or your work is so stressful that it sucks away the time and energy you would otherwise have to take care of yourself.

Or you may believe that you don't have the resources you need: You feel that a lack of money, not having a good personal trainer, or not knowing how to cook is stopping you from reaching your goals. On NBC's hit television show *The Biggest Loser,* overweight contestants compete to lose weight by going to a ranch where they have around-the-clock access to a state-of-the-art gym, personal trainers, a medical team, and deliciously prepared foods. You may feel that if you don't have circumstances as conducive to weight loss as they are on the ranch, you can't be successful.

I CAN'T

Finally, Resisting Responsibility means that you may place blame on a perceived personal shortcoming—something you believe to be an unchangeable characteristic that stands between you and weight-loss success. You feel *trapped* in an overweight body, afraid that yo-yo dieting has ruined your metabolism and that no amount of exercise can help. You have cravings and give in to eating unhealthy foods when others seem to be able to resist. Thoughts and attitudes such as these rob you of confidence in your ability to make and stick to changes, as well as confidence that those changes will make a difference for you.

CHAPTER 9

The Willpower Myth

Definition: A belief that those who are successful at losing weight possess an innate power to do something that they really don't want to do and stick with it for the long run.

Undermining Thought: "What's wrong with me? I was doing great and now all I can think about is chocolate torte with raspberry sauce. Argh! If I only had more willpower, this diet would be a breeze."

The Willpower Myth Quiz

1. I am good at following rules. If someone will just tell me exactly what I need to do to lose weight, I know that I can do it. Yes/No

2. Losing weight is *very* important to me, so I have to wake up each day ready to do whatever it takes. Yes/No

3. I feel stupid or inadequate when I fall off of a popular diet because it should be easy to follow when the rules are spelled out so clearly. Yes/No

4. Posting a picture of myself at my heaviest weight on the refrigerator will make me stay away from after-dinner snacks. Yes/No

5. I typically start off strong on a diet program, but after a while I lose interest. Yes/No

6. I know exercise is good for me, but I just can't make myself do it consistently. Yes/No

7. I often give in to tempting foods and feel like I should have better control over myself. Yes/No

8. I really want to reach my goal weight, but I'm just not very motivated to change my diet or start exercising. Yes/No

9. I feel like losing weight should be easier for me because I want it so badly. Yes/No

10. I have been in a diet and exercise "zone" where nothing tempts me to cheat or veer off course. I know I can get back there. Yes/No

WHY WILLPOWER IS A MYTH

If you've ever followed a diet plan before, you've probably swung between the extremes of total excitement and complete lack of motivation. It can happen over a few days or weeks or it can happen in an instant, when the waiter wheels the dessert cart to your table.

The biggest problem with willpower is that, well . . . it doesn't exist in the way you may think. Willpower is generally defined as the ability to control one's actions, impulses, or emotions. That sounds real enough, and the hope that it exists in a way that will help you lose weight is so desirable and appealing that it rivals the appeal of the Fountain of Youth. But, sadly, willpower is about as likely to show up when you really need it as that fabled fountain is to begin spouting right in your backyard.

Willpower is nothing more than a very strong, internal motivation; it's the same motivation you get anytime you really want something and are willing to do the work it takes to get it. The obstacle here is believing (a) that willpower is a trait that you either have or don't have and (b) that willpower alone will enable you to do something that you are not ready to do, or for which you lack the necessary skills.

STRENGTH WON'T COME WITHOUT DESIRE

You may have noticed that your willpower is at its strongest when you are eating healthy and exercising. But it will most likely abandon you when you're struggling and need it most. This sudden "loss of willpower" may leave you feeling inadequate and wounded.

It might sound absurd for us to tell you that you might not be ready to lose weight. Of course you want to lose weight! But wanting the weight to be gone and being willing to truly change your lifestyle and put in the work to lose it are two very different things. It's quite possible that you're not ready to take on the challenges of making healthy changes and you're relying on willpower to help you overcome your resistance. But if you've never given much thought to what motivates you to lose weight, beyond the number on the scale—which proves time and again to be too weak a motivator to keep "dieters" engaged in healthy behaviors—or you don't possess the skills necessary to navigate the ups and downs of real life, no amount of willpower will help. It is flawed thinking to believe that if you just "try harder" you will eventually succeed. Rather, it is more likely that the frustration will continue and, in time, you will quit entirely.

Relying on willpower as a cornerstone of your weight-loss program is a critical mistake. And popular diets that tempt you with amazing before and after pictures while serving up extremely rigid rules only feed the Willpower Myth. They make you believe that you *should* be able to achieve the same results if you only set your mind to it and that you *could* do it if you wanted it badly enough.

CHAPTER 10

Tuning Out

Definition: Not listening to the signals from your body and mind.

Undermining Thought: "I am a meal skipper. I'm just not ever that hungry. I don't need to eat 1,400 calories a day."

Tuning Out Quiz

1. I expect exercise to be painful, and I know I need to push through it. Yes/No

2. I rarely feel hungry. Yes/No

3. I often eat until I'm stuffed. Yes/No

4. I often skip meals and end up feeling incredibly hungry in the afternoon or early evening. Yes/No

5. I don't sleep well and usually consume more than one caffeinated beverage each day to help me get my work done. Yes/No

6. When I feel discomfort while exercising, I don't know whether I need to back off or push harder. Yes/No

7. I feel like I am doing great with my diet if I can make it through the day without eating much. Yes/No

8. When my body hurts, I routinely take medicine for the pain so that I don't have to slow down. Yes/No

9. I like to go, go, go, and I often feel resentful or frustrated that I don't have more energy. Yes/No

10. I frequently go to sleep too late and feel exhausted the next day. Yes/No

IS YOUR ENGINE LIGHT ON?

Imagine driving a car without knowing that something urgently needed servicing, or even whether your gas tank was nearly empty. Without the dashboard indicators, your car might still function and get you where you were going. In fact, it might seem just fine right up until the moment it stopped dead on you.

You may be treating your body like an old car. You ignore what is really going on inside, hoping that the knocking under the hood will just go away on its own. You walk around unaware of feeling hungry or thirsty, just as likely to go all day and "forget" to eat as to eat a whole sleeve of cookies without remembering a single bite. You go without sleep and stay at work until you're completely exhausted but you sit on the couch all weekend because you're too lethargic to move. When you exercise, you may quit at the first sign of a sore muscle, or you may push through the pain and end up with a serious injury.

I'VE GOT TO GET AWAY!

It's understandable that people need to tune out some of the mayhem in today's fast-paced culture. We are bombarded with news and information, work stress, family challenges, and financial worries, and our mental well-being depends on being able to filter out those things that don't require our immediate attention. However, tuning out from what your *body* is telling you will lead to poor health decisions. Your body's natural signals (like hunger, fatigue, and pain) get progressively more difficult to hear amid the buzz created by caffeine, alcohol, sugar, fat, and medications. Eventually those natural signals may disappear altogether; they might still be there beneath the surface, but because you've spent so much time ignoring or suppressing them, you've lost the ability to detect them. And underneath it all, health problems are brewing. As the health problems worsen, new signals—such as reflux, low blood sugar, or painful, swollen joints—emerge. These are symptoms of disease or injury, and they'll be much harder to ignore.

TUNING OUT LEADS TO A DIET MENTALITY

These more serious signs that something is wrong may eventually wake you up and trigger your desire to change. But, after years of Tuning Out, you have lost your ability to recognize the natural signs of hunger and fatigue.

Some cultures have traditional and very natural ways of listening to hunger signals and heeding them to prevent overindulgence. Okinawans have a traditional eating practice called harahachibu, which means eating until you are about 80 percent full. But Tuning Out means ignoring these signals until it's impossible to notice when you're satisfied or starving. Likewise, Tuning Out strips away your natural ability to feel how much movement is good for you. Now that walking as a mode of transportation and manual labor are both largely absent from our lives, we've lost a degree of connection with our bodies that used to let us know when we were doing too much.

With your ability to hear your natural signals so diminished, you have little choice but to rely on external rules, such as strict diets and exercise regimens, to help you make basic, healthy choices. This means you resort to severe calorie restriction and denial of any pleasure from food. And you exercise just to burn more calories and end up going overboard in pursuit of "fixing" your body rather than rejoicing in how it feels to move.

CHAPTER 11

Selective Accountability

Definition: Picking and choosing which aspects of your weight-loss program you want to follow or keep track of and to whom you will be accountable.

Undermining Thought: "I can do well during the week and write down every bite I eat. But my weekends are different—my schedule is so crazy that I don't eat very healthfully and I don't have time to write it all down."

Selective Accountability Quiz

1. When I set a goal, I don't like to change it—even when a change in circumstances has made it unrealistic to accomplish. Yes/No

2. I am good at tracking my progress when I am doing well. Yes/No

3. If I am not diligently following my diet and exercise plan or the number on the scale isn't dropping, I make up excuses to cancel appointments with my personal trainer, nutritionist, walking partner, or anyone else who might be supporting me. Yes/No

4. I tend to set my goals too high because I would be embarrassed disclosing goals I feel are "easy" to reach Yes/No

5. I find it hard to "practice what I preach." I can tell others how to successfully lose weight, but I find it hard to stick to the plan myself. Yes/No

6. I like to set goals in areas in which I am doing well, and I don't like to focus on the areas in which I struggle. Yes/No

7. I can't stand disappointing others. If I don't reach a goal, my first thought is of how I'm letting down my friends and family. Yes/No

8. If I've had a tough week, I stop tracking and journaling and forget about my goals until things settle down. Yes/No

9. I prefer to have impressive goals and like it when others get excited by them. Yes/No

10. When I come up short of my goals, instead of looking for a way to do better the next week, I usually feel deflated and beaten down. Yes/No

MAKING A GOOD IMPRESSION

When we discuss accountability in this section, it refers to your being accountable to a professional (a coach, personal trainer, nutritionist, therapist, or doctor), or to friends and family, or to yourself (through tracking and journaling). A person who is being selectively accountable is happy to be accountable for the areas in which he or she is making progress but covers up the areas in which there is a problem. You may know someone at work who makes sure word gets around when he does something great. But he might avoid challenging situations, such as spearheading a new project, where he risks coming up short. Or he may dodge his fair share of responsibility, letting others take the rap when a project isn't going well.

Similarly, in the areas where things are going great with your weight-loss program, you are more than ready to review your progress and talk about the next steps. However, in the areas where you are struggling, you want to avoid accountability altogether. For example, you may highlight how well you are managing breakfast, but you don't deal with the problems you have with late-night snacking.

EXPECTATIONS AND ACCOUNTABILITY ARE CONNECTED

On the surface, Selective Accountability might seem like a simple on-again, off-again attention to detail that could easily be remedied. But it's likely that the reasons for Selective Accountability run deeper than that and stem from having unrealistic expectations, not wanting to disappoint yourself or others, and using denial to help minimize any feelings of failure.

If you are superexcited to get in shape, clean up your diet, and see significant—even dramatic—weight-loss results, you're putting a lot of pressure on yourself to perform. These expectations may be based more on what you *wish* would happen and the results you'd *love* to see than on what you are currently capable of doing consistently.

Going back to the example of the workplace, setting extremely high expectations is like overpromising to your boss what you can realistically deliver before a deadline. It is human nature to want to impress those to whom you are accountable. But by setting expectations that are *too* high, you only increase the chances that you will face failure and disappointment.

And when you do come up short of your weight-loss goals, Selective Accountability actually pushes you away from communicating with those who are there to help and guide you. You are upset with yourself, maybe even ashamed of your actions, and you worry about disappointing others or having to deal with any "judgment." To avoid the disappointment, you skip meetings and stop writing down your updates, tracking your goals, and even thinking about your program.

SLIPPING INTO DENIAL

Finally, Selective Accountability can put you in denial about the reasons why you are not reaching your goal. You may not see clearly how Selective Accountability thwarts your progress. You can't understand why you aren't losing weight because you feel like you are doing well by tracking *most* of your exercise and eating and meeting *many* of your goals. The gaps in your reporting, however, offset consistent weight loss and lead you to believe that you are not able to lose weight despite doing "everything right."

PART 3

THE FIVE STEPPING-STONES TO CHANGE

A wareness of what is holding you back is an important part of being able to move forward. But, now that you have had a chance to think about the mental roadblocks you have been facing in your weight-loss efforts, it's time to begin the next part of your journey. The Stepping-Stones are five powerful ways of thinking that can decrease or remove the power that your obstacles have over you. As your thinking in each of these five areas evolves, you will find that the Seven Undermining Obstacles to Weight Loss have less impact on your life. While there is not a one-to-one relationship—one Stepping-Stone is not designed to "fix" one particular obstacle—you will recognize elements within a particular Stepping-Stone or a series of Stepping-Stones that do tie directly to an obstacle and will help you overcome it.

The first three Stepping-Stones—Expecting Greatness, Regaining Your Balance, and Creating Successful Environments—help set the stage for the final two, Being Unstoppable and Awakening Your Intuition. What you'll learn in "Being Unstoppable" (see page 82) is vital to maintaining your healthy lifestyle when life becomes challenging, and in "Awakening Your Intuition" (see page 97) you'll learn how to tune in to your feelings and use your senses to help you make healthier choices. However, because some areas of your thinking may need more work than others, feel free to skip around and focus on those areas that are most relevant and meaningful to you.

To help you progress through each Stepping-Stone, we have broken them down into three "thinking shifts" that we consistently observe in our clients as they move toward a full understanding of that Stepping-Stone. And you will find an "A-Ha" Exercise at the end of each thinking shift. These will help you practice the new concepts, approaches, and ways of thinking that we introduced in the preceding section.

We have included real-life success stories from some of our clients throughout the Stepping-Stone chapters (see "I'm Coaching Myself Thin!" on the following pages). As you get to know these men and women, you'll see how a specific Stepping-Stone has been instrumental in helping them achieve real and lasting weight loss.

I'm Coaching Myself Thin!

MEET THE PEOPLE MAKING IT HAPPEN

The quotes and stories in the following chapters were shared with us by a few of the terrific people we have worked with. We have chosen examples that characterize the kinds of changes you will make on your own journey to a healthier life and lasting weight loss.

We will introduce each client here by describing the formidable obstacles he or she faced when starting out, as well as the turning point when each decided to make lifestyle changes. Throughout the next five chapters, we'll provide quotes from each client relevant to the shifts we are describing.

Jenifer

AGE: **36**

HEIGHT: **5'6"**

OCCUPATION: **Accountant**

HEAVIEST WEIGHT: **250 pounds**

CURRENT WEIGHT: **176 pounds**

BEGAN HER JOURNEY WITH US: **2006**

Obstacles: Jen was completely sedentary and her weight was creeping higher. She resorted to extreme measures to lose weight. "I'd scale back on calories as much as possible and cut out anything I considered junk food for a while, but then would slide right back to old habits." Even though she knew that her diet strategy wasn't working, she didn't know what to do. "I used to hate myself, was miserable, and dealt with a lot of my depression by eating. I built up walls. I'd act like I didn't care, but I was hurting inside." Jen used food to cover up her feelings of unworthiness in a futile cycle that only magnified those feelings.

Turning Point: In 2006, Jen found herself topping out the doctor office scale at 250 pounds. "My dad had just had two cardiac stents and had been diagnosed with diabetes. I was scared that I might be headed down the same road," says Jen.

Joyce

AGE: **68**

HEIGHT: **5'8"**

OCCUPATION: **Retired CPA**

HEAVIEST WEIGHT: **210 pounds**

CURRENT WEIGHT: **137 pounds**

BEGAN HER JOURNEY WITH US: **2007**

Obstacles: Joyce was an old-school dieter. She tried every diet pill (even amphetamines when they were legal) to help her slim down. She was all about the quick fix because she didn't know there was another way.

Turning Point: "I was so tired of not being able to keep up with my husband, and I hated how stiff and sore I'd feel when I tried to get out of the car," says Joyce. She decided it was time to take an honest look at her relationship to food, exercise, and weight loss.

Roxann

AGE: **53**

HEIGHT: **5'9"**

OCCUPATION: **Software Implementation**

HEAVIEST WEIGHT: **370 pounds**

CURRENT WEIGHT: **220 pounds**

BEGAN HER JOURNEY WITH US: **2007**

Obstacles: Roxann had been yo-yo dieting for most of her life. "I'd lose 100 pounds on an ultra-restrictive diet of my own making, and then I'd gain 150 back—and I did this more than once," she says. She traveled extensively for work and didn't know how to live healthy while on the road and living out of hotel rooms.

Turning Point: On New Year's Eve 2005, Roxann's husband, Steve, was rushed in to the ER with throat constriction, and even though he turned out to be fine, Roxann answered yes to every risk factor question that was asked of Steve. It scared her terribly, and she cried the entire night. And the next day, there was a *Biggest Loser* marathon on TV.

Ryan

AGE: **35**

HEIGHT: **5'5"**

OCCUPATION: **Graduate Student**

HEAVIEST WEIGHT: **287 pounds**

CURRENT WEIGHT: **205 pounds**

BEGAN HIS JOURNEY WITH US: **2011**

Obstacles: Ryan struggled with weight for years and didn't think he had the strength or willpower to succeed. He had people around him telling him that he couldn't do it.

Turning Point: After turning on *The Biggest Loser* show, Ryan realized that people really were losing the weight, getting healthy, and keeping it off. He said, "I started to think that I don't want to be 35 years old and be on blood pressure medication and on the fast track to diabetes. I wanted to be able to run, ride my bike, and live a long and healthy life, no matter how difficult it was, because I saw that it gets easier."

Renee

AGE: **36**

HEIGHT: **5'3"**

OCCUPATION: **Controls Engineer**

HEAVIEST WEIGHT: **270 pounds**

CURRENT WEIGHT: **142 pounds**

BEGAN HER JOURNEY WITH US: **2007**

Obstacles: "In my senior year of high school, I was cut from the soccer team, and it killed my chances of playing in college—and was a huge blow to my self-esteem," says Renee. "That's pretty much when my weight issues began. It really changed the whole trajectory of my life," says Renee. "Dieting was on my mind every day—I was either dieting or pigging out in the anticipation of a diet that I'd be starting tomorrow. I always felt bad about my weight, and I was always panicked because it kept going up. After I lost the weight—I was sort of stuck on using exercise to maintain my weight. The first year I did Jazzercise to maintain. I think I did 600 classes in a year. I'd do two or three, sometimes four, classes in a day. It was insane."

Turning Point: Even while she was stuck in her All-or-Nothing Thinking, she knew that it wasn't the way. "I knew what Michael and Greg were teaching was different—but I was still using a lot of my old diet rules. I knew I had to break myself of all of this."

Tricia

AGE: **41**

HEIGHT: **5'5"**

OCCUPATION: **Schoolteacher**

HEAVIEST WEIGHT: **170 pounds**

CURRENT WEIGHT: **138 pounds**

BEGAN HER JOURNEY WITH US: **2007**

Obstacles: Tricia had been using the same All-or-Nothing diet strategy for years, but it wasn't working. "I'd cut out sweets and snacks and eat three small meals. I'd go full force, reach my goal, and then I was done. I would snack on whatever. If the kids ate something—I'd finish whatever they left over. If I wanted a snack, I'd grab them from the cupboard. You know I'd buy the cookies for the kids' lunches—but then I'd eat them."

Turning Point: On her last diet, Tricia lost 10 pounds, and then in 6 months she had gained 20. That was the final straw for her. She stepped on her bathroom scale and saw 170—her highest ever. "My size 14s were tight, and it dawned on me that at this rate, I am going to be over 200 in no time!"

Steven**

AGE: **42**

HEIGHT: **5'9"**

OCCUPATION: **Financial Management**

HEAVIEST WEIGHT: **253 pounds**

CURRENT WEIGHT: **216 pounds**

BEGAN HIS JOURNEY WITH US: **2010**

Obstacles: Steven didn't make his health needs a high priority and his past weight-loss efforts came up short largely because he expected faster results. He would undereat and battle hunger as well as struggle with consistency given his busy travel schedule for work.

Turning Point: Steven's grandmother pleaded with him to make changes. She had already buried a husband and a son and didn't want to bury a grandson as well. He is very close to her, and he promised that he would start doing something about it. In addition, he had reached a point that he also wanted his clothes to fit better and to be more attractive to his wife. He wanted to build up his confidence in order to finally get the promotion and raise he felt like he'd earned at work. And he knew he would have to find a plan that he could adapt to his needs, one that would work for him despite the hours and travel that his work requires.

**Name has been changed

CHAPTER 12

Expecting Greatness

Lewis Carroll said "If you don't know where you are going, any road will take you there." The problem is that "there" on your weight-loss journey may not be a place where you are thinner or healthier. Without a detailed road map of where you want to go, you may try to get some-where, only to end up right back where you started. Sure, you probably have a specific goal weight or number on the scale in mind, but what you may fail to realize is that losing weight is the means to, not the end of, your journey.

And what is there at the end, exactly, besides a number? What, exactly, do you expect once you reach that long-coveted number?

When pressed to specify what you will get for your dieting efforts, you might respond with something along the lines of "toned up," "feel better," or "have more energy."

Do these vague aims give you direction? Truly inspire you? Doubtful.

It turns out that the goal of losing a particular amount of weight isn't really motivational at all. If it were, our country wouldn't have the prob-lem with obesity that we currently face. What this goal does do is put unbearable pressure on you to lose a specific amount of weight in a short period of time. Weigh-ins become judgment day for whether your plan is "working" or not. What you are left with are some very high expectations for what you have to do to be successful, without a vision of what that suc-cess can mean to you.

Expecting Greatness means, you will need to bring to bear both a healthy dose of realism and an expansive imagination. When it comes to changing your behavior, these qualities are an excellent and complemen-tary combination. Being realistic about how much you can exercise per day, which nutrition changes to make gradually, and how fast you will lose weight opens the door to the possibility of sticking to a beneficial eating and exercise plan for the rest of your life.

With the power to stick to your healthy behaviors comes the ability to improve many other aspects of your life, including relationships, career, travel opportunities, sports, hobbies, and your general sense of independence and confidence. This is where the expansive imagination comes in. Instead of being completely dependent on weight loss for all of your motivation, imagination helps you consider a world of possibilities and be excited by them. You will find, perhaps much sooner than you thought, that great experiences are waiting for you, and that the possibility for even greater ones will pull you into action. You will move toward your goals because you want to, instead of feeling that you are forcing yourself to do them.

THINKING SHIFT: LEARN TO BELIEVE IN CHANGE

The diet and exercise industry has been feeding you a lie: They want you to believe that real change is made only by people who have the "right" plan or the "best" exercise equipment—whatever it is they are currently trying to sell. This ploy can make you want to buy their ideas or products, whether you have a plan to actually use them or not. You see companies' slim, fit, confident spokespeople, and when you assess how far you are from achieving what they have, change begins to look about as possible as your winning the lottery.

The fact is, you can't expect greatness when you're constantly doubting whether the plan you're on is the right one or the best one. If you're worried that some other approach might work better or you're suspicious that you're not doing "enough" to lose weight, you're setting yourself up for failure from the start. Plus, this constant distrust of yourself can quickly spiral into the excuse that you can't change without some sort of magic bullet. If you just didn't have to go to work, if you could exercise with that famous trainer, hire a great chef, or attend that renowned weight-loss program, *then* maybe you could be successful.

Because the myth that there is a "best" way to lose weight is so ingrained in our culture, your tolerance for a plan not working is likely to be quite low. After a few days of not losing weight as fast as you'd like, or as fast as you've been told to expect, you're probably looking for what to try next.

Believing in change, then, means believing that the plan you are on *will* work. The good news is that what does work is not as complicated as you might think!

Throw out all of the fad diets, the influence of politics and big business on dietary recommendations, and the endless debates about which kinds of food cause us to gain weight. The basic message about what constitutes healthy nutrition has been the same for decades: Eat more fruits and vegetables and whole grains. Limit refined grains, saturated fats, and added sugars. It's really that simple.

If you ignore all the hype about which exercise is the best or burns the most fat the fastest, you'll find that the guidelines on physical activity could simply say: Do some moderately intense activity most days of the week. Do errands. Lift and carry things. Limit your time in front of the computer and TV.

And there is no best "fat-burning" workout. The type of exercise that is best for you is the one you will keep doing consistently. If water exercise is what is right for you or what you enjoy, then it doesn't matter if running burns more calories per minute. If you're not ready to begin strength training, it's fine to begin with "just" walking.

When you look back in 10 years, chances are that this core advice about nutrition and exercise will not have changed very much. What this means for you is that you can follow the very basic guidelines we give you in *Coach Yourself Thin,* avoid the lure of the next "new" diet or exercise gimmick, and relax about whether you're doing things "right."

Have Faith in You

Believing in change means believing that *you* are capable of change. People just like you change their lives for good every day. It is not necessary to be full of self-confidence right from the start, because successes early on breed more success moving forward. And from there, confidence can grow. Therefore, you must adjust your expectations to make sure they are realistic. This will allow you to experience success right from the start.

Commit to the Task at Hand

Imagine yourself at your goal weight, and you may see your whole life changing. You'll see yourself as happier, more energetic, and more successful,

I'm Coaching Myself Thin!
BELIEVING IN CHANGE

Jen: "When I began to understand and believe that I could really stick with *this* plan, I realized that I had crossed the line from just *another diet* to actually making permanent changes I wanted to keep forever," Jen says. "I used to think that there was either 'on the wagon' or off, but now I know that there is no wagon at all."

Ryan: "The first step and one of the most important steps to being successful is believing in the path you're on and giving up trying to find shortcuts. I recall the moment I realized that the only thing that would work was healthy eating and exercise. After this shift, I started to lose weight without feeling tired."

Roxann: "I had spent so many years on so many different diets that I was superskeptical about anything working for me. While eating real food versus following a restrictive plan looked good, food-wise, I hated the idea of eating more frequent meals and snacks; it sounded crazy. I kept looking for a flaw or a gimmick—something to make it fail—but the suggestions were simple (like grilling meat instead of frying it, and eating mostly whole foods), and it was less expensive than other plans I had tried, so it seemed doable."

and this image will convince you of how important your weight loss is. What may be less obvious is that to change for good, you'll need to accept that the *means* to achieving that weight loss is important, too.

In today's culture, it's easy to believe that you don't need to eat healthy foods in healthy portions in order to lose weight. If you believe the advertising, you can reach your weight-loss goals by simply turning to weight-loss supplements or a fad diet.

It's also tempting to believe that you don't need to exercise to lose weight. Calorie restriction is a very effective tool all by itself. And some "healthy" weight-loss plans downplay or ignore the need to exercise at all—some even use the lack of a big commitment to physical activity as a selling point.

Given the opportunity to simply wake up at their goal weight, most people would probably opt to skip the work to get there. Unfortunately, even if a miracle occurred and you were suddenly a size 6, you wouldn't stay that size for long. The fact is, any miracle weight-loss solution is bound to fail because it won't give you the skills needed to keep the weight off in the future.

Did you know that a person taken straight from sea level to the top of Mount Everest would die within minutes? Yet the summit has been reached over 2,000 times! Climbers train their bodies by hiking to base camp and living there for several weeks, then making trips to progressively higher camps along their route. Continuing to descend back to lower camps allows their bodies to recuperate and adapt to the demands of the altitude before making that final ascent.

This is a good analogy for weight loss: Repeatedly climbing and descending the lower slopes of the mountain is the work you must do to develop the strength to reach the summit, and no amount of being "fired up" about summiting Everest—or losing weight—will help you if you don't do the necessary work to get there. Embracing the tools of change is vital to your success.

To sustain your effort, the work itself needs to be something you enjoy to some extent. If the work is pure sacrifice, the desire to do it will end, no matter how sweet the reward. While some of the tools and strategies we suggest (such as writing down everything you eat in a day) won't be necessary forever, embrace them now in order to make changes that will last a lifetime. You can make it easier on yourself by making the work fun; use an inspiring journal to log your food and exercise, try an app on your phone, join an exercise class or walking group, or build a recipe collection to share with your health-minded friends.

"A-Ha" Exercise

Baby Steps Exercise: Identify one behavior that you believe is important for you to change in order to improve your health and begin your weight-loss journey. Choose something you think will make a noticeable improvement in an area of your life in the next day or two, such as by increasing your energy, letting you sleep better, or boosting your confidence. Then assess your ability to follow through using this scale:

I believe in my ability to [*insert specific goal*].

1. Strongly disagree

2. Disagree

3. Neither disagree nor agree

4. Agree

5. Strongly agree

If you answer at a level of 3 or below, choose a different behavior. Examples:

Drink four 8-ounce glasses of water each day.

Eat two servings of fruit and three servings of vegetables each day.

Walk outside for 10 minutes each day.

Go to bed 30 minutes earlier than normal each night.

Commit to making this change for the next 3 days. After 3 days, answer the following questions:

How successful were you in practicing this behavior?

How did this behavior affect your health?

How did this exercise help you believe you can make healthy changes?

THINKING SHIFT: REDEFINE SUCCESS

We understand the allure of achieving a sought-after number on the scale. This fascination with achieving certain numbers and milestones is everywhere today. A lot of people think that happiness means making a certain salary, owning a certain car, or living in a particular neighborhood. Yet the satisfaction of a material purchase is short-lived. Similarly, in our experience, a number on a scale cannot make a person happy, at least not beyond the initial joy of having reached it. You can aim with all of your might to lose 200 pounds or 10 pounds, reach that goal, and feel no different than you do today. The magic that number seems to hold simply evaporates the closer you get to it. The genuine joy you experience when you first reach a weight milestone is significant, but the fact that reaching your goal weight isn't life changing can be disconcerting enough to knock you off track and send your weight immediately upward again.

One of the most powerful thinking shifts you can make is widening your view of what constitutes success. Accept that you need to count on something other than the scale to prove that your life is changing. When you do, you begin to own your lifestyle change as it occurs rather than waiting until you hit your goal weight to feel good about your achievements. You

I'm Coaching Myself Thin!
REDEFINE SUCCESS

Tricia: "I had been weighing myself every day, but I'm not doing that anymore. It is not all about the scale. It is about how I am feeling and my energy level. I am already seeing some other changes. My abs are tighter from strength training and I noticed that my arms were sore, so I know I am challenging my body. It's funny because I used to hate to sweat. I was a real anti-sweat girl, but now I like to sweat and even stink—it means I really pushed myself today. That's success."

Ryan: "The first thing that motivated me was that I ran 2 miles without stopping. It was dusk and sprinkling out so my friend and I were the only two on the track that night. I made it all eight laps and from that moment on, I knew that if I'd done it once I could always do it. Now I'm ready for a 10-K. It just takes a little proof to yourself that you can do something and the *impossible* becomes quite possible."

Joyce: "At 67 years old, I can now do things that I never thought I could do. I strength-train and now have defined leg, calf, and arm muscles. Growing up as an overweight child, I didn't know I could get those! I can lift things, and my back, hips, and knees don't bother me like they used to. Getting up and down has gotten so much easier, too, thanks to doing squats. I want to keep up with my adult daughter and my 16-year-old granddaughter. On her last visit, my granddaughter exercised with me every day."

relate to what it's like to live your life in a healthy and active way, leaving your "fat" clothes and "fat" way of thinking behind you.

You can expand your idea of what success means by being conscious of what we call "nonscale victories," or NSVs. These victories can be emotional, physical, or spiritual. They can be related to any aspect of your life, including but not limited to food, activity, stress reduction, self-esteem, relationships, and career, as well as your ability to be physically independent and feel capable and confident as you navigate the world around you. NSVs can be as simple as enjoying the taste of fresh fruit or making a new friend in your exercise class. They can be as practical as being able to use the lap belt on an airplane or fit into a theater seat. And they can be as meaningful as learning to turn on some music instead of reaching for food when you're feeling stressed, or realizing that you're not ashamed to go swimming. When life gets in the way of your weight-loss plans and you need to remember why it is well worth your efforts to continue down your path to health, think of all the NSVs you would not have achieved had you not started down this road to begin with.

If You Had "Three Wishes"

It may sound melodramatic, but NSVs can help you live a life you have only imagined. Perhaps your weight has held you back from going out with friends, asking someone on a date, being intimate with your partner, going to museums or movies or plays, traveling, playing sports, asking for a promotion, going back to school, enjoying the beach or an amusement park, or going to the gym or pool. Feeling confident enough to do any one of these things can be nothing short of dramatic.

At the beginning of this journey, chances are good that you simply wanted to lose weight for the sake of seeing a particular number on the scale, but eventually it will be about so much more. An interesting parallel can be drawn between how losing weight and spending money can add meaning and happiness to your life. Specifically, research has shown that, in some cases, having money to spend can indeed make you happier. However, it's not the amount you have to spend but what you spend it on that matters. The type of purchase most associated with adding value to your life is one that you can *do* something with. Spending money on experiences or things that allow you to have experiences (such as vacations, recreational and sports equipment, or theater tickets) increases your happiness more than buying something like a fancy watch does.

And we have seen this same phenomenon in our clients: It's not the amount of weight they lose but what they choose to do with that weight loss that matters. Our advice to you, then, is to stop thinking about being a particular weight and start thinking about what being your current weight is keeping you from *doing*. Travel, recreation, wearing nice clothes, being more romantic—all of these experiences will be richer and more enjoyable if you are fit, confident, and full of energy. In that way, having your health is like having money to spend on things that make you happy. The more capable you are of enjoying these activities and experiences without losing your breath or being embarrassed, the more likely you are to go out and live. The success of living the way you want to will surpass anything the scale can tell you and can withstand any attempt by the scale to take that success away. We want you to know this up front. Knowing from the outset that this reward can be yours can help you "get over the hump" of wanting just the weight loss. Once you do that, it will feel as though you have been granted three wishes for a healthier life!

"A-Ha" Exercise

Nonscale Victories (NSV) Exercise: The true test of an NSV is that you consider a change a victory even when the scale does not show a loss. This exercise works best if you weigh yourself once a week or once every 2 weeks, on the same day. Right before you step on the scale, reflect on the last week or two and write down three to five NSVs you've noticed. How does identifying your NSVs change your reaction to the number on the scale? Is it helpful for you to acknowledge yourself for your efforts and identify signs of progress *before* stepping on the scale?

Keep an updated list of NSVs posted in a prominent place or write them down in your journal so you can easily revisit them at a later time.

THINKING SHIFT: EXPAND YOUR VISION

The Quick Fix Mindset has trained you to want big changes in your weight and to believe that you can see those changes quickly. Our clients often tell us, "I *need* to see weight-loss results or I won't stay motivated." Talk about a self-fulfilling prophecy!

As we mentioned above, making healthy lifestyle changes rests, in large part, on being able to adjust your expectations in a way that will allow you to experience success early and often.

If you are given a task that you see as completely insurmountable, you will soon find yourself feeling paralyzed. Diets that require you to follow complicated regimens or completely give up your favorite foods will frustrate you to the point of quitting, as will exercise plans that are too strenuous for your ability level or that demand too much of your time. But you cannot simply lower your expectations to increase your motivation.

For example, you might understand that switching to a policy of not "drinking your calories" is an important step toward losing weight, but you might not feel that this step alone is worth pursuing because it's not a strict regimen. Similarly, you might understand that all movement burns calories, but you might not really believe that walking 5 minutes at a time during your work breaks is enough to matter. In both of these cases, the goal doesn't feel worthwhile because it's not designed to take the weight off quickly. But if that attitude keeps you from doing anything at all, then it's hurting your chances of ever making healthy changes. One of our clients, Tricia, used to blow off the 40-minute workouts she'd scheduled for herself because she never had the time; with four kids and a preschool teaching schedule, 40 minutes just wasn't realistic for her. But Tricia soon realized that doing a 20-minute workout was better than not working out at all!

In order for you to embrace your weight-loss journey, you must take steps that are small enough to achieve on a daily basis but large enough for you to feel the promise of progress and success in your efforts. Your steps must help you evolve, not leap, toward goals that are increasingly challenging and rewarding. This is how you stay in the Motivation Zone.

Finding Your Personal Motivation Zone

At the beginning of this chapter, we pointed out that most people have not defined what they expect to get out of losing weight beyond something mundane and uninspiring, such as to "tone up," "feel better," or "have more energy." And that lack of vision, combined with the high expectations we just discussed, sets you up for a lose-lose scenario.

But you can turn it around. The realistic expectations discussed above are just half of the equation—a personal, powerful, and expansive vision is the other. Set your sights beyond weight loss; focus on what your life can become as you become more fit and healthy. What will your new life look like? What exciting things will you be capable of doing? What places will you visit? As your vision of what you want for yourself becomes more expansive, your ability to take on more work to achieve that life becomes greater.

A strong, personal, meaningful vision of the life you want creates more resolve on your part to achieve it. It gives you a road map for success and wings to fly with, instead of a cross to bear.

"A-Ha" Exercise

Vision Exercise: Visualize yourself having a great day. See yourself smiling and being genuinely happy as you greet your family, co-workers, and random people on the street. Imagine saying hello to a stranger, letting

I'm Coaching Myself Thin!

EXPAND YOUR VISION

Roxann: At the end of her first year with us, Roxann had lost 123 pounds, and she maintains a 150-pound weight loss today. She has competed in many races with her online friends, and her confidence has excelled at her workplace. "It was extremely important that I started living before I lost all the weight," says Roxann of her first 5-K. "I was 280 pounds, but I finished the 5-K in under an hour." Roxann was happily surprised that most athletes were very welcoming of her despite her size.

Jen: Jen discovered that small steps lead to bigger challenges. Once Jen had mastered running and healthier eating and the weight was coming off, she had a major confidence boost. She went on to get her MBA with a 4.0 average!

Renee: "Fortunately, my inner athlete came back when the weight started coming off. Early on, I was proud of performing a hike that was rated 'difficult' in Red Rock Canyon with some of my friends. Then I quickly turned to races. I've had many victories: my first 5-K, 10-K, triathlon, half-marathon, marathon, half-Ironman, and all the way to my first Ironman! And the not-so-sensational motivators really keep me going, too, such as being able to get down on the floor and play with my crawling nieces and nephew, or having the energy to chase them around the yard as they've gotten older. I'm even going to start coaching soccer for my niece's team. If I'd been asked before, I wouldn't have had the confidence in myself or the energy to do it."

someone merge onto the freeway, holding the elevator door for the delivery guy, and cooperating on a project at work. Consider all kinds of ideas for what you can do to have a great day.

Next, pick a day to put your vision into action. Throughout the day, write down everything you do to make your day a great one and how each action affects how your day turns out.

How did it help you to "see" the vision of having a great day ahead of time?

CHAPTER 13

Regaining Your Balance

When you think about finding more balance in your busy life, you may think, "Well, maybe if I were a monk somewhere in a monastery, with nothing to do but eat, sleep, and meditate, I could *finally* feel balanced." But since you're probably not a practicing monk, it's likely that you have a very full schedule that requires prioritizing and planning if you're going to make it all fit.

The fact is that your life today is extremely demanding. An imbalance arises anytime you get too little sleep, consume too much food, or are plagued with stress. Add to these everyday challenges the need to manage relationships, work obligations, family time, and expenses, and it is no wonder that you struggle to make it all work.

To achieve balanced eating and exercise, you must overcome cultural pressures to have and do it all. On one hand, you are told that you can look like the beautiful models on magazine covers, and on the other hand, you are being urged to "supersize" your fast-food meal. The media sells you equipment and programs to develop six-pack abs, but it also encourages you to spend your evenings watching reality TV. Ads for "energy beverages" promise that you can manage fatigue well enough by using caffeine to help you get through the day. And as the subtle signs of underlying imbalances become more serious health problems (like acid reflux, insomnia, or constipation), you reach for the many over-the-counter and prescription medications that help you manage their symptoms. The Quick Fix Mindset makes you question why you should have to give up your favorite chili dogs when you can just take an antacid an hour before you go to the ball game.

If you imagine a wide rushing river and think of the strong current as the direction we are being pushed in as a society, you can visualize how easy it is to get swept into certain habits and behaviors—to just go with the flow. After all, you go along feeling like you are just living a "normal" life and doing what everyone else is doing, and then one day you wake up wondering how your good health disappeared. It was an effortless ride, and in all fairness, it may have been an exhilarating one—but now you want to push back against the current and get your life and well-being back.

If you can recognize what in your life is out of balance, then you have taken the first step toward reclaiming your health. You may realize that you have been eating too much junk food, and as a result, you've gained weight and feel sluggish. Or perhaps you make the connection that a lack of exercise or activity each day is the reason you're severely out of breath when you take the stairs.

The next step is to take a healthy approach—rather than a Quick Fix one—to feeling better. What you are about to discover is that living a "healthy" life is not as complicated as you have been led to believe. It's really pretty basic once you toss out the fads and hype. You can learn to recognize a good, practical diet and exercise plan and not fall victim to false promises any longer.

In all likelihood, you will need to paddle consistently against a very strong current if you are going to move in a new direction. At first, paddling upstream is hard work. But as you find your balance and your own personal rhythm, seeking out and using what works for you as you pursue a healthy life, it will get easier.

THINKING SHIFT: DEMYSTIFY "HEALTHY"

The redeeming quality of a diet is that it provides structure, but most of the diets out there are flawed because they are too structured. Most diets require you to follow a set of restrictions and rigid rules that are not livable because they mean you have to put your normal life on hold. As convincing as a weight-loss book may be when it spells out what you should and should not do to be successful, the truth is that there is no one-size-fits-all weight-loss plan—and restriction and sacrifice are not the name of the game.

A balanced plan should be expansive, increasing the variety in your diet. It should encourage you to be active in whatever ways you can and want to be, rather than demanding that you perform a particular brand of superintense, magically slimming exercise. A balanced plan is manageable from the start and designed to improve your chances of success, not undermine those chances by recommending drastic changes to your diet and exercise.

The Basics of Healthy

You are very likely confused about what a balanced diet and exercise plan should look like, and it's no wonder: All of the plans seem to contradict each other about what is healthy, and passionate debates rage on over whether animal products, fruits, and grains are good for you or not and whether there is a best way to exercise to lose weight. For now, forget about finding any consensus.

Let's focus on key points that can help you achieve balance with your diet and exercise. In Parts 4 and 5, we'll elaborate on the points below and help you create a healthy, working plan.

Nutrition

Here are four simple guidelines to help you feel better and get on a healthy track right from the start.

- **Stay hydrated.** Drink at least 48 ounces of water or until your urine is clear or light in color, which is a reliable measure of hydration status.

- **Eat enough.** You need to eat enough quality calories each day (see Part 4 for a specific calorie goal) to support your bodily functions and metabolism. Drop below your calorie goal, and it will actually become more difficult to lose weight. Plus, when you eat enough you will feel better and have more energy for exercise.

- **Balance your intake.** Eat consistently throughout the day to help balance your blood sugar levels and keep your appetite in check. Find the right balance of carbohydrates, protein, and fats at your meals and snacks to feel satisfied and control cravings.

- **Eat mostly whole foods.** Stick with the evidence—there is an overwhelming consensus that *whole food*—all-natural meats, seafood, dairy products, whole grains, nuts and seeds, beans, vegetables, and fruits—are the key to a healthy diet.

I'm Coaching Myself Thin!

DEMYSTIFY HEALTHY

Renee: "One of the first things I learned was that I needed to eat more. This went against the grain of what I'd thought before. I had been starving myself, and I had to learn that this never lasted. It was a big change. I had also been constantly starting a diet. So, I'd starve myself for one day—or half a day—and then I'd blow it. And I'd go back to eating my junk food. I'd eat practically nothing one day, and then I'd binge the next day. My body was so mixed up. I had to learn to eat more frequent meals and snacks. That was not my style. It's kind of funny; the better I've gotten at eating healthy, I realized that I was avoiding good carbohydrates, complex carbohydrates, because of old diet thinking. It hit me one day: Wow, I could eat a sweet potato and that would be good for an endurance athlete."

Tricia: "I wasn't quite sure how I was going to follow the eating plan recommended by the Biggest Loser Club. It said to eat cereals, pasta, and other carbohydrates, and I had been doing the whole low-carbohydrates thing. Thankfully, Greg helped me learn the difference between healthy carbohydrates and unhealthy ones, and he taught me to eat smaller meals throughout the day and to modify meals to make them work for my whole family. I started by adding fruits and vegetables to each meal. So instead of spaghetti, sauce, and bread, we'd have spaghetti, sauce, salad, and fruit. Today, I faithfully add fruits and vegetables to all our meals."

Joyce: The first thing Joyce learned from us was that all her previous diet extremes were destined to fail. She would keep weight off for 1 to 3 years, and then quickly regain it. "Whereas I used to try to eat the least amount of calories possible, I now know to eat the right amount of healthy calories," she says. "I never realized that fiber was an essential part of a healthy weight-loss or maintenance eating plan. Now I know that if I get protein and fiber in my meals and snacks, I'll stay satisfied for longer."

Activity

Here are four tenets of any healthy exercise program. Keep them in mind as you design your own exercise plan in Part 5.

- **Keep it simple.** Stick to basic exercises that you already know how to do or that are easy to do, and start out at a level that feels comfortable to you.

- **Form follows function (and genetics).** To change the way your body looks, you have to change what your body is capable of doing. But genetics also contribute to your shape. Therefore, aim to be the best you that you can be and stop comparing yourself to supermodels and world-class athletes.

- **Listen to your body.** If it hurts, stop. If you feel winded or sick, take a break. If you feel like you can go a bit harder, give it a try!

- **Make it fun.** If your activity feels more like play, you're more likely to do it. Improving your fitness is a terrific way to achieve non-scale victories. If your fitness helps you do other things you value, such as walking through a park or playing with your children, it will become more important to you.

It will take some trial and error to find the diet and exercise approaches that work best for your body and your lifestyle. And while those particular approaches may change over time, the basic values behind them will remain unchanged.

"A-Ha" Exercise

Myth-Buster Exercise: Read a magazine article on weight loss or watch a dieting infomercial. Write about the aspects of the article or ad that are misleading, such as the promised rate of weight loss or the "magic" exercises or foods that will supposedly make losing weight easy.

How has believing these claims interfered with your ability to stick with a healthy and sustainable program? How have you been affected by weight-loss myths in the past?

For the coming week, become a weight-loss myth-buster. Keep your eyes and ears open for weight-loss–related myths in the media, and write them down in a place that you will see daily.

How does being on the lookout for myths help you change your own thinking about weight loss?

THINKING SHIFT: FIND YOUR BALANCE POINT

As we discussed earlier in this chapter, the demands of today's culture have a tendency to pull you out of balance and push you toward being overweight, overworked, stressed-out, and in need of caffeine and/or medication to make it through the day and past the pain. Whatever your personal work or family situation may be, chances are that you are busy from the moment you wake up until the moment you go to sleep at night. And the odds are good that you feel like you need to be *on* at every turn. There just isn't enough time or energy to eat right or get to the gym regularly, much less time to journal or pamper yourself. And given the expense of raising a family today, there may not be enough money to buy more fruits and vegetables or to belong to the gym in the first place.

To stand any chance of defeating these obstacles to better health, you will have to paddle upstream against a strong current. But you can reclaim your time, energy, money, and life in the process. This shift relies on your being able to see what good health offers you: the opportunity to feel and look good and to have the energy and vitality to do things you currently can't.

Protect Your "Me Time"

Many people say that they don't have time to exercise or fix a healthy meal. While that might feel true to them, it's not really the case. We all have the same amount of time in a day, and we all tend to do the things we deem most important. You need to recognize that time spent improving your health is as important as time spent on other daily tasks.

There are many things you can do to carve out time to take care of yourself and to nurture and sustain your health. You can shift your schedule, delegate tasks, ask for help, and cut out or cut down on television and computer time. In order to become healthier and weigh less, you must find a way to prioritize the behaviors that will help you reach those goals. You may have to overcome the notion that "me time" is inherently selfish; taking care of your health is one of the most selfless things you can do. If you are committed to being the best parent, partner, friend, or caretaker you can be, then spending the extra time to improve your health creates a win-win situation for you and your loved ones.

One caveat when it comes to "me time" is that it doesn't always have to be spent alone. Prioritizing more quality time to strengthen your relationship with your spouse or your kids is certainly nurturing and beneficial.

I'm Coaching Myself Thin!

FIND YOUR BALANCE POINT

Roxann: "In the past, I'd park as close to work as possible and, even then, I'd be wheezing so hard I'd have to duck in the lobby bathroom, wash my face, catch my breath, and do whatever I needed to become composed enough to take the elevator. It was that hard to move. Then I began to exercise by parking as far away from work as I could and just walking. I would take my time but still get out of breath. Soon I realized, 'Hey, I'm not out of breath anymore and I've made it all the way into the clinic.' I noticed that just this little bit of activity was starting to help with the weight loss."

Tricia: "I realize now that what works this week won't necessarily work next week. There might be an assembly at one of the kids' schools, but being flexible is the key. Before, I would just throw in the towel when my schedule got crunched. But now I think, Okay, what can we do as a family that might be active?"

Learn from Your Past

When it comes to weight loss, you can learn a lot from what has and has not worked for you in the past. A good way to assess what *has* worked is to look at the behaviors and strategies that you held on to the longest, perhaps even to this day. Maybe you know that the only way you can fit in exercise is if you do it before work. Maybe you find it very easy to eat a healthy breakfast, as long as you have the ingredients you need in the house. As you prepare to make changes this time around, include those positive discoveries in your plan.

On the other side of the coin, think about what failed you when it came to losing weight in the past. Did your plan require you to eat a lot of foods you dislike or demand a tremendous amount of time for cooking, shopping, and planning? Did it rely on gimmicky strategies that you grew tired of, such as consuming energy bars or other meal replacements to help you make it through the day? Did the workout plan seem too hard or too easy, or did it require equipment or facilities that you don't have easy access to?

The true test of whether a plan is workable is trying to imagine whether you could still be following the eating guidelines and the exercise plan a year from now. If the answer is no, then don't bother with it. Find something that feels manageable, right from the start, and build from there. Parts 4 and 5 provide the guidance you'll need to get on track.

Stop Putting Your Health on "Credit"!

When you notice the difference in price between a fast-food hamburger and a serving of high-quality chicken or beef, or between a large bag of chips and a head of broccoli, you may think that you can't afford to eat healthy foods. The long-term truth, however, is that you can't afford *not* to spend more money on your health right now. Think about it in terms of "pay now, or pay later with interest." The costs incurred later in life are not just financial—they're measured in terms of physical pain, illness, and loss of abilities. The costs also include lost time spent with your children or grandchildren. And financially speaking, investing in your health today will help you save thousands of dollars in the coming years by avoiding costly over-the-counter and prescription medications.

You may also find that leading a healthier life will cut other nonfood-related costs immediately. Cutting down on your TV time may mean that you can reduce the cost of or even eliminate your cable package. Depending on where you live, you may be able to get to work under your own power, by walking or riding a bicycle. Maybe you will be able to stop buying pain relievers, antacids, and sleep aids. You could eliminate the cost of soft drinks and avoid costly vending machines, convenience store stops, and $4 coffees. And if you decide to eat out less often and cook more meals at home, the savings can be even greater.

The truth is, your "conveniences" are costing you more—both in dollars and cents and in your future health—than making healthy choices ever will.

"A-Ha" Exercise

King or Queen for a Day: Come up with a plan to treat yourself like royalty for at least a few hours, enlisting friends or family as needed to help you make it happen. Do something out of the ordinary for yourself: Get a massage or a pedicure, take a luxurious bubble bath with candles, request your breakfast in bed, take a quiet walk in a park, or schedule a golf outing.

Describe all of the feelings you experienced while planning and following through with your personal time.

How would occasionally taking the time to nurture yourself like this help you in your weight-loss journey?

Write down three ways you plan to nurture yourself during the coming month.

THINKING SHIFT: LET GO OF PERFECTION

Have you ever completely sworn off your favorite junk foods or started an exercise program with the intention of running or walking every single day, only to see your dedication fizzle in a matter of a few weeks—or less? When it comes to losing weight, there is no doubt that big changes need to be made, but why set the bar so high and in such an extreme way?

Blame it on the Quick Fix Mindset and the influence of a culture that sells you *perfectionism* every time you look at an airbrushed model. Parents inadvertently teach their children to strive for perfection, whether it's with school attendance, athletic success, or maintaining a perfect report card. As an adult, you try to keep a spotless house, do everything right at work, and go the extra mile to be attractive.

In all fairness, there is a place for perfectionism and unrelenting precision—heart surgeons and astronauts come to mind. And there is nothing wrong with aiming to excel in most areas of your life. But, in our view, there is a difference between striving for your best and trying to be perfect. When you strive to do or be your best, you leave room for mistakes and learning. Even heart surgeons and astronauts allow themselves a learning curve as they prepare for an actual operation or mission. But living a healthy life takes place in an ever-changing environment. The learning never stops, and there is no "mission" that you need to perform flawlessly. Adhering to rigid rules for the sake of weight loss is just an attempt to apply the laws of perfection to your environment and yourself. And attempts at "perfect" weight loss are doomed to fail miserably.

"Most of the Time" Is Enough

Perfectionist thinking would have you believe that you are either *on* or *off* of your program. You'd view foods and behaviors as either good or bad, with good foods and behaviors causing you to lose weight and bad foods and behaviors leading to weight struggle or weight gain. Perfectionism doesn't make room for real life to occur; it doesn't allow for those everyday situations that knock you off track. These events are a normal part of life, and if your plan doesn't allow you to adapt—to exercise less when you're pressed for time, have an extra treat now and then, eat out occasionally—your forward progress and your motivation will come to a grinding halt. Try as you might, you'll never stick to any plan 100 percent of the time. And things fall apart quickly when coming up short makes you feel like a failure.

That means that the path to success is moderation in your very approach to change. You need to accept that it is okay to make healthy choices "most of the time." Success literally depends on your understanding that not only do you not have to be perfect to reach your goals, but that aiming for perfection sets you up to fail.

Defining the 80/20 Approach

One balanced approach to lifestyle change is the 80/20 model. The idea is that 80 percent of your choices are made in the planned and predictable environment of your "normal" routine and are therefore mostly healthy, while 20 percent of your decisions are made in situations that are not part of your normal routine, and therefore may include indulgences or lapses. You might be at a birthday party and have a slice of cake, or maybe you get superbusy at work and miss a few days of exercise.

At first glance, an all-or-nothing approach actually seems easier to stick to because it's so black and white; there are hard-and-fast rules that are simple to follow. The 80/20 approach, on the other hand, requires judgment and moderation; you have to make decisions and choices on the fly. For example, can you have just one of your trigger foods (one of those foods that you struggle to eat in moderation) in a given situation? Can you take a day off from exercise and get right back to the gym the next day?

The keys to making 80/20 work are that 1) understanding that the 20 percent is a normal part of life and it's better to make peace with it than attempt to avoid it altogether, and 2) you haven't "blown it" and one indulgence or lapse doesn't have to cascade into several more.

Bringing Moderation to Life

What you use your 20 percent for is a very individual decision, and you must be selective about what is important to you and what is not. You might decide to indulge in an unexpected treat that doesn't necessarily fit into your plan for the day—a margarita at a festive social event, a favorite dessert at a local restaurant, or a unique bottle of wine opened by a friend. On the fitness side, you may skip your workout because some friends call you up at the last minute to go out, and it just sounds too fun to pass up.

In some cases, the 20 percent could be a true slip, rather than an intentional choice. Maybe you neither intended nor truly wanted the food or the day off from exercise: Your self-control truly failed you, or time got away from you before the gym closed. It will happen. But the 80/20 model helps you see that a small slip is inconsequential as long as your healthy 80 percent is there for you.

The 80/20 approach is not as exciting as trying to follow an extreme plan because it does not promise speedy, extreme weight loss. However, it will give you something that has been missing from your previous efforts: lasting results. Once you break free of All-or-Nothing Thinking (see page 22) and allow yourself to splurge on special occasions as *part* of your weight-loss program, you can relax and empower yourself to have long-term success.

When you say yes to 80/20, you are saying yes to:

- Living without fear of indulging on special occasions.
- Letting go of guilt after the occasional indulgence.
- Having a structure that offers guidance, but also flexibility to modify your plans as your life changes.
- Managing lapses by keeping them in perspective, learning from them, and moving forward (rather than dwelling on them, punishing yourself, and giving up completely).
- Living a sustainable lifestyle and having a greater chance of sticking with your program.

"A-Ha" Exercise

80/20 Exercise: Think about a previous weight-loss program you tried, and identify two areas where you strove for perfection and set extreme goals. How long were you able to stick to the program?

If you rewrote those goals to include ranges that move away from perfection, such as "I will walk 4 or 5 days this week instead of aiming to exercise on all 7 days," or "I will limit myself to three or fewer sodas this week instead of trying to cut out soda altogether," how do you think this would have affected your success rate?

How does it feel to "lower the bar" for what you expect from yourself?

Think of one health-related goal you can commit to for the coming month. Write it down, ensuring that it is moderate and includes some flexibility.

At the end of each week, write in your journal about how being flexible affected your ability to stick to your goal.

I'm Coaching Myself Thin!

LET GO OF PERFECTION

Renee: "In the past, I was a total perfectionist. If I got something wrong in the middle of the day, I'd blow the whole rest of the day. Now, I find room for little splurges and never feel deprived. It is the first time I have ever felt I had 'enough' while losing weight, and I truly feel this mental shift toward 80/20 thinking is what carried me through the duration."

Roxann: "Learning to be less than perfect took a lot of practice. I realized that I'd been too strict and that I really had to find a way to make *not perfect* a part of my life. I discovered that I can eat what everyone else is eating in the right amount, with a few modifications, and still lose weight. I have to live my life."

Joyce: "I am a bit of a perfectionist. I always think I should do a little more, lose a little more, exercise a little more. It's something I have to work at, but I don't think that I'm the all-or-nothing person I used to be either. When it comes to letting go, I like to have treats around the house. If a candy bowl is there, it is a choice, and I trust myself to make the choice. When I see that bowl, I reflect on where I am during the day and whether I really want it and can fit it in, and then I can make a conscious decision."

CHAPTER 14

Creating Successful Environments

A typical busy day can illustrate how your environment can control your ability to make healthy choices. Your co-worker brings in a package of your favorite chocolate chip muffins and asks if you would like one; you glance over at the front desk and see that the candy jar has been filled again with peanut M&Ms; and then you realize that there is a lunchtime presentation today that is catered, which means an oversize sandwich, a bag of chips, and a cookie. When you get home that night, you just don't see the point in saying no to the pecan praline ice cream when your spouse pulls it from the freezer. And forget exercise: You sat at your desk all day, and because there aren't any safe places to walk in your neighborhood, you don't feel very comfortable going for a stroll after dinner.

If this is how your day looks, it's no mystery why you're struggling. You just don't feel like you have that much control over yourself or your environment. However, it is very likely that feeling out of control is more of a perception than a reality. No one actually forces you to eat anything unhealthy or to stay glued to your chair throughout the day. Lack of planning, work stress, and feelings of obligation and responsibility (or perhaps a reluctance to make other people angry or uncomfortable) all contribute to these perceptions. But you have more control than you might imagine.

THINKING SHIFT: MAKE "HEALTHY" EASIER

Wouldn't it be easier to resist the call of pecan praline ice cream if you had to drive to the supermarket when the urge for it hit? The Law of

Displacement refers to the notion that if you decrease the availability of or limit your access to unhealthy options, you will begin to think of them less often. Conversely, if you add healthier choices to key areas of your environment, you'll think of and choose them more often. Using this strategy will eliminate the vast majority of your unhealthy eating that happens simply because the temptation is there and you reach for it on a whim.

The first displacement strategy is Omission. This means completely eliminating the unhealthy choice from your environment: Out of sight, out of mind. What processed, sugar- and fat-laden snacks can you simply toss? Obviously, there may need to be a good deal of compromise with family members who may not be quite ready to give up all of their treats. You might start by asking them what snack food they most want you to buy. If you negotiate this change by offering to leave some snacks in the house but have them prioritize their favorites, they are more likely to cooperate, and you'll still end up with fewer unhealthy options in your kitchen. You may be surprised to find that your children start eating more of your healthy snacks when given the opportunity.

The second displacement strategy is Line of Sight: putting the healthy choices out where you can see them and hiding the unhealthy ones, or just making sure that you don't see the unhealthy ones. Stick the candy jar on the top shelf of the cupboard and put a bowl of fruit in the middle of the kitchen table. Change your route home to avoid the bakery, or take the scenic route to the bathroom at work to avoid passing the break room. And take the TV out of the kitchen so you don't see all of those tempting food ads while you're preparing and eating your healthy meals.

Did You Know?

Whether it's the candy dish at work, the appetizers at a social function, or the peanuts you snack on while making dinner, absent-minded eating can easily amount to between 400 and 800 calories a day and be the explanation for weight gain or difficulties with weight loss. A variety of strategies can help you raise your awareness and reduce the frequency of amnesia eating. (See Hunger and Fullness Scale on page 135 and "Tune In to Your Mind" on page 104 for examples.)

The final displacement strategy is Substitution: replacing an unhealthy choice with healthy ones. You may well be able to resist the muffins in the break room when you have a low-fat Greek yogurt and low-fat granola in the fridge, or you might decide to bring a pear and a whole foods–based energy bar to displace the chips and cookie that come with the catered lunch. You can engage in calorie-burning activities instead of sedentary ones when possible, such as by walking up the stairs to your office instead of taking the elevator. At home, we highly recommend replacing large serving dishes with smaller ones so you'll have the opportunity to tune in to your fullness cues before you add more food to your plate.

Streamline Your Changes

When you are trying to eat better and exercise more as part of a hectic, anxiety-ridden schedule, it is essential that you are able to make lifestyle changes as efficiently as possible. Do a little extra now to help you save time later. For instance, you might make larger portions for dinner and freeze the extras so you have quick and healthy meals for another day. Or you might put chopped veggies in a bag for tomorrow's snacks while you make your salad for dinner. Keep a running grocery list of your healthy food essentials—the fruits, vegetables, snacks, high-fiber cereals, and other staples that you must have in the house to stay on track. Also, keep a stash of healthy canned goods (like tuna) and a favorite lower-sodium soup in your pantry. Keep frozen chicken and vegetables in your freezer so you can always pull together a quick and healthy meal.

If meal variety is important to you, you may need to widen your repertoire of simple, healthy recipes and learn the cooking skills needed to create them. This may be as easy as getting a couple of cookbooks for making quick and healthy meals or just buying a few new spices or other condiments.

When it comes to exercise, think about turning your work breaks into opportunities to get in some movement. By going to the restroom and water fountain at the far end of the building, you take a mental break and get in a short walk at the same time. Also, keep your exercise clothes in a gym bag at the foot of your bed, so you're always ready to grab it and go.

I'm Coaching Myself Thin!
MAKING HEALTHY EASIER

Roxann: Roxann has learned to speak up for herself. If her team at work is planning a late dinner meeting, she lets them know she'll need some downtime beforehand to take a walk, get a healthy snack, and map out the restaurant menu (she often looks online to find appropriate options). In restaurants, she's quick to remove the bread basket, ask for vegetables instead of French fries, and have the waiter preportion half her entrée into a to-go box. "The most grief I get is for asking for a full pitcher of water, but if it is there I know I'll drink it," she says.

Steven: "I have put my foot down at work: I do not accept 7:00 a.m. meetings anymore. I work for a global company and time zones are a problem, but I do not need to sacrifice my life. With this one change, I have ensured I can work out before I get the day kicked off. Once the day starts, it's easy to find 1,000 reasons not to do the activities you need to do to stay active."

And when you come back from a workout, make it a habit to exchange the clothes you've just used with clean replacements.

Work on ways to make your exercise time more efficient. Do you find yourself wandering around at the gym, wondering what to do next? You could book a session with a personal trainer who can teach you how to design and execute an effective workout. Explore exercise class options at your gym and keep an updated schedule handy. If you don't have a gym membership, build a library of favorite exercise DVDs so you always have a convenient, go-to workout that you know you'll enjoy. Or scout out exercise possibilities near your house, such as a walking route through your neighborhood. You may be lucky enough to live near a park with athletic fields, basketball courts, walking and running paths, a "fitness trail," or even paddle boats. Use online resources and local parks and recreation departments, and check class listings at gyms and community centers. Be prepared: It can take a while to develop a healthier routine, but rest assured that if you stick with it, you will soon learn how to make your exercise sessions take up less of your day.

Focusing your attention on being as efficient as possible will not only create more space in your day, it will also introduce you to the concept of "plugging your time drains." Who knew that you spent 15 minutes staring at the 24-hour news channel when you walk in the door from work? Isn't the 5-minute wait for the elevator just enough time to walk up the stairs to your office? Join a gym that is between your office and your home so that you can stop by on the way to or from work. Do the same with grocery shopping: Find a market that has an excellent produce selection and that you pass on your way home. Two or three quick stops there each week will increase the likelihood that you'll always have fresh fruits and vegetables on hand.

Finally, think about how you really want to spend your precious downtime. Watching a movie you've been dying to see, reading a compelling book, listening to music, writing in your journal, or doing some light yoga might be more relaxing and nurturing than watching television, paying bills, or surfing the Internet.

"A-Ha" Exercise

Law of Displacement: Pick one of the three displacement strategies (Omission, Line of Sight, or Substitution) and think about a specific way that you can implement it today. You may decide *not* to bring home a trigger food, such as chips; take a tempting tin of cookies off of the countertop and put it in a cupboard; or replace a salty, processed afternoon snack with yogurt and fruit.

Make the change today and follow through with it for the next 3 days. At the end of that time, write down any thoughts you have about how this change did or did not benefit you. Include these changes as part of your healthy eating goals (see Part 6) for the coming month.

THINKING SHIFT: DISCOVER YOUR "INNER CIRCLE"

When you start overhauling your lifestyle, attitude, food preferences, and exercise habits, your family, friends, and co-workers will witness these changes and there will likely be some reaction. Some will turn out to be your most reliable supporters, others will remain neutral, and—unfortunately—some will undermine your efforts with either resistance or outright sabotage. By resistance, we mean "push back," an unwillingness or inability to be supportive and facilitative of the changes you're making. By sabotage, we mean a conscious attempt to undermine your progress.

Resistance occurs when those around you neglect to take your healthy lifestyle into account. They may not be interested in making healthy changes or they may have their own ideas of how to go about dieting and exercising. Either way, they don't want your choices to change their daily routines, pressure them into exercising with you, or affect their ability to eat what they want. Co-workers may continue bringing doughnuts to the office. Your spouse might bring home takeout from a restaurant you are trying to avoid, even though you've fixed a healthy dinner. Your kids might clamor for unhealthy snacks that you happen to find tempting, too. And instead of the great family hiking trips you may have pictured, you might find yourself leaving everyone at home while you go exercise alone.

Saboteurs, on the other hand, will take these scenarios one step further by *deliberately* putting obstacles in your way. For example, a co-worker who brings doughnuts to the office might put one on your desk or ask you repeatedly why you won't have just one. Or your spouse might urge you to "go off your diet for a night" and go out to one of your old haunts. Your family might complain and make you feel guilty about how long it takes to get dinner on the table when you have to go for a walk first. And you will encounter criticism: You may hear that your efforts to live healthier are silly, fruitless, or selfish.

Managing the Fallout

You will probably feel disappointed when you realize that you cannot count on all of your family and close friends for support. But the truth is, you don't need *everyone* to be supportive for you to continue pursuing your goals. In the following sections we cover strategies you can use to manage resistance and sabotage.

Speaking Up for Yourself

As the Bible says, "Ask, and it will be given to you; seek, and you will find; knock, and it will be opened to you." (Matthew 7:7) When you face situations that may compromise your weight-loss efforts, you may have an all-or-nothing tendency to want to either avoid the problem entirely or give in completely. Society has conditioned you to give away your power: You may be convinced that your needs are not important and that you shouldn't make any waves "just" so you can take care of yourself. However, you can do a lot more than you realize by putting your foot down on your own behalf. The more you ask in a powerful yet tactful way for the help and support you need in order to live a healthier life, the greater the possibility that you will receive it. In the process, you will inspire others by your determination and willingness to go the extra mile for yourself. If your health is a priority to you, it's important to speak up, just as you would if it were the health of a loved one that you needed to attend to. For example, if your commute cuts into your time to work out or cook a healthy dinner, ask your boss if you can change your work hours to avoid heavy traffic. Speak up about the junk food served at staff meetings. If you brought in a fruit bowl, put it in a prominent place in the office, and hid the candy jar in a cabinet, would your co-workers complain or applaud?

Ask friends about changing where you hang out after work. Choose restaurants with fresh, healthy food choices, and order sparkling water between mixed drinks to deflect attention from the fact that you aren't drinking as much alcohol. Let your friends at work know that you will be using several of your lunch hours each week to go for a walk, and ask if anyone would like to join you. Look for windows of opportunity to spend time with friends who might share your interest in being healthier. Together, find things to do that you can enjoy without being tempted to make unhealthy choices. (See the "A-Ha" Exercise on page 78 for more information on spending time with people who are more supportive.)

If you encounter resistance (which you might, at first), be assertive. And if resistance persists, remember that you have the ability to limit your time with certain friends and coworkers. There are circumstances where you don't need to tell others what you are doing or why. Many of your friendships, especially the more casual ones, will be better maintained if you keep the details of your healthy lifestyle changes to yourself. Only talk about what you really need to in order to get through those situations where staying silent jeopardizes your health. Avoid trying to make converts of anyone; rather, let your actions speak louder than your words. If people are interested, they will come and talk to you to learn more about the changes you have made.

The Art of Compromise

With your close friends and family, it is still necessary to speak up for yourself and ask for what you need. Asking for help keeping junk food out of sight or finding the time to fit in exercise is just as important at home as it is at the office or with casual acquaintances. The biggest difference between work and home is that you are less able to (and typically don't desire to) limit the time you spend around close family and friends. This is where compromise comes into play.

Let's say you and a close friend have a routine of meeting for margaritas, chips and salsa, and a hearty Mexican meal twice a month. You've always really looked forward to being able to splurge and let off some steam, but you know now that this meal would knock you right off your healthy track. You may consider giving in and continuing your routine to avoid awkwardness, or you may avoid her or make up excuses for why you can't go. Ultimately, either path could jeopardize the friendship: the first because you'd blame her for your lack of success and the second because you'd create distance between the two of you.

If you truly value her friendship, the more positive path to take is to openly ask for what you need. Tell her that you are very serious about your efforts to lose weight and you can't afford the temptation right now, and then ask if she would be interested in changing your get-togethers to an activity that didn't involve food. Ideally, this suggestion will open up a whole new array of activities for the two of you to do together and make the splurges a thing of the past. Her answer may be that she wants to compromise and do something active sometimes but still go out for Mexican other times. In that case, you've still cut down on the temptation you'll face and you can look at the meals with her as opportunities to practice your restaurant eating strategies (see page 127).

When it comes to your family, let's say they like to hang out and do nothing on Saturday mornings. You enjoy the downtime together, but you find that it leads to overeating because breakfast seems to go on for hours. Plus, you end up feeling lethargic for hours afterward. In this case, you could suggest that you all go to the park to ride bikes, go for a walk, or play a game together. Or perhaps your family wants to compromise and you agree that after the park you will take them to a local restaurant—one where you know you can make healthy choices—so that nobody has cooking to do or dishes to clean.

Of course, even with close family and friends, there is the chance that compromise simply won't work. In these cases, one suggestion is that you compose a letter to your friend or family member stating exactly what you need in order to be successful and why it's important to you (see page 233). If directness and assertiveness don't work, then consider seeking outside assistance with the relationship. See the Resources on page 273 for help finding a professional counselor.

Build Your Support Network

It is possible to proactively cultivate your own weight-loss support network: a group of people that you can count on to brainstorm solutions and celebrate victories with you. Start by taking an inventory of your family, friends, and co-workers; identify those individuals whom you can count on to be openly, unconditionally supportive of your healthy lifestyle. These should be people who have shown you from the start that they are genuinely happy that you're taking better care of yourself. You can rely on them to support you, practically and emotionally; go out of their way to help you find healthy places to eat; go for a walk with you; reassure you when your confidence is low; and celebrate with you when you succeed. This group of people will become your "inner circle," and they will help you overcome any obstacles in your path. Think of it as putting a safety net in place: They'll help keep you from falling too far or being off track for too long.

After you've recruited family members and friends to your "inner circle," consider the sources of support that you are aware of in your community: fitness groups, such as walking, hiking, or cycling clubs, as well as groups that are sources for fresh, locally grown foods, such as food co-ops or farms that offer community supported agriculture (CSA) plans. Check out community bulletin boards and weekly newspapers that list events and gatherings. You are likely to find support groups on a variety of topics, including weight loss. Attending these meetings is an excellent way to meet new people on the same lifestyle track as you, as well as a great way to gather new ideas.

Group exercise classes at your gym, local yoga studio, or community center may be offered for a small fee or even included with your membership. These classes provide you with quality instruction and are probably organized by skill or conditioning level to ensure that your exercise is safe and effective. Think about taking a cooking class, too, perhaps through a local market that specializes in fresh, healthy ingredients.

Web sites can provide a wealth of information, as well. Subscribe to a weight-loss site that offers daily support for a reasonable monthly fee, or start your own support group on a social networking site like Facebook. One of the biggest benefits of belonging to an online community is that it allows you to give support to and get support, at any time of the day or night, from other people who are going through the same lifestyle changes as you. Blogging and message boards are excellent tools for reaching out to your support network whenever you want to celebrate a victory or you need a hand.

Finally, there are health professionals in your community who can offer support: medical doctors, behavioral and physical therapists, personal trainers, dietitians, and wellness coaches. For one-on-one care to evaluate illness, injuries, exercise form, and behavioral and emotional issues related to your health and weight loss, or even to provide external motivation when you really need it, the services that these professionals can provide is unparalleled and irreplaceable. (*Note:* Because wellness coaches typically provide their services via the telephone and Internet, that field is an exception to the necessity of being face-to-face.) Think about reaching out to members of this professional community whenever you feel stuck in your progress or have a health issue that you are unable to find answers for on your own. The monetary cost is much higher than for online communities and resources, but the peace of mind can be worth every penny.

"A-Ha" Exercise

Bull's-Eye Exercise: To differentiate between supporters, nonsupporters, and saboteurs in your life, draw two large circles on a sheet of paper, one inside the other, to create three separate spaces in which to write the names of people in your life. In the inner ring, list the people that you know you can count on to support you in any situation. In the middle ring, list the people who you don't think you can count on for support but who you don't believe will offer resistance or sabotage you. And in the outermost space, list the people who are likely to stand in the way of your success by resisting your efforts or by putting obstacles and temptations in your way.

Think about ways to increase or maintain your interactions with your inner circle. What can you do to nurture these relationships?

Think about ways to keep people in the middle circle in a neutral

I'm Coaching Myself Thin!
DISCOVER YOUR INNER CIRCLE

Joyce: Joyce finds that staying balanced means staying in touch with her wide network of support, which begins with her husband and constant companion, Frank. They have several ways of exercising and having fun together, including the post office walk, Wii Fit games and videos, and a little hiking. "I also make sure to stay active when my 16-year-old granddaughter comes to visit. We play games and exercise videos," says Joyce.

Roxann: "When I perused some of the message boards on the Biggest Loser Club, I started seeing some really cool interactions between people who had never met face-to-face. And it sort of came to me all of a sudden: I wasn't utilizing any support systems at all. In the past, I'd leave behind all support once I lost some weight because I thought I was 'there' and I didn't need any help. Now I could see that I'd never stop needing help, and I started believing that support was part of the key to change. Now my main support is my Foxy Ladies, my online support group through the Biggest Loser Club. These women motivate me constantly. I wouldn't have kept off more than 150 pounds without them."

place. How might you open the door for them to have more negative influence over your health decisions, and how can you keep that from occurring? Are there people in your middle circle that you believe would respond positively if you were to invite them to join you in your healthy lifestyle? If so, consider reaching out to them.

Divide the people in your outermost circle into two categories: close friends and family, and casual friends and extended family. Limit the time you spend with people who are not close friends or family, and follow the suggestions in "The Art of Compromise" (see page 76) to help deal with close friends or family in your outer circle.

THINKING SHIFT: USE CREATIVE FLEXIBILITY

Despite making major changes to your environment and developing a solid support team, you may face unexpected obstacles as you navigate constantly changing surroundings, expectations, and responsibilities.

Imagine going through a major job change. You're now working in a different office building on the other side of town, and your longer commute greatly cuts into your exercise time and your morning routine of packing a healthy lunch and snacks. The change in location has completely eliminated your chance to shop at your favorite whole foods market on your drive home. Plus, your responsibilities in this new job are different: You're expected to meet with clients over lunch or dinner, and the meetings are scheduled at the last moment. All of a sudden, many of your strategies for fitting exercise into your schedule and planning out your meals and snacks have been completely upended.

Adaptability

Perhaps, up until now, such a scenario would have been more than enough to knock you off track. But, as you have become more thoughtful and proactive in creating a nurturing environment and building a support network, you have noticed a shift in your attitude. Now you are more determined not to let your program fall by the wayside. Here are some examples of win-win ways to become more adaptable.

A Creative Commuting Solution

You realize that since your commute home takes you a full 50 minutes during rush hour, going straight to the gym near your new office after work and then driving home once the traffic has diminished is the simplest, most rewarding way to fit in a workout every day and still get home in time to cook a healthy dinner. This may require you to change gyms, but the health benefits will far outweigh the financial cost or short-term hassle of making the switch.

Surviving an Unexpected Lunch

You show up for work to discover that a lunch meeting has been called, and you know what to expect from the catered meal: roast beef or turkey sandwiches, potato salad or chips, a big chocolate chip cookie, and a soda. You need a game plan so this meeting doesn't derail your healthy eating for the day. Fortunately, you brought a low-fat yogurt and an apple for your afternoon snack. (You had been planning on grabbing soup for lunch.) You decide to eat half of the catered turkey sandwich, replace the chips and cookie with your healthier snacks, and stick with bottled water from the break room. You have successfully navigated a lunch that would have been disastrous in the past.

"A-Ha" Exercise

Creative Solutions Exercise: Identify an area of your life where it feels like you have little or no control. Brainstorm several ways that you could modify the situation to help you gain more control. What changes to your schedule would work wonders for fitting in healthy meals or exercise? Consider tools that could help you make healthier eating and exercise choices, such as an insulated lunchbox that you can fill with a nutritious meal for work or a pair of comfortable shoes that you could wear to walk the stairs during your lunch break. Find a co-worker with similar interests and create a weekly healthy eating and exercise challenge that will help you both stay more focused at work. Write down and commit to trying at least three of your brainstorming ideas.

I'm Coaching Myself Thin!
USE CREATIVE FLEXIBILITY

Ryan: "The first challenge I really had was at Christmas this past year. I was returning home to visit my mother, and I knew it was going to be challenging, as she always makes a bunch of cookies and our traditional holiday dinner is made in the good old southern style: lots of butter and sugar. I allowed myself one cookie a couple of times while I was there and told my mother that I was going to cook Christmas dinner as a gift to her. I made her traditional dinner with substitutions for the butter and sugar and everyone loved it. They had no idea I'd changed anything. When it came to dessert, I made her traditional desserts and just ate my normal evening snack of yogurt with granola and dark chocolate chips for my dessert."

Steven: "The most creative thing I did was change my drinking habits on business trips. My favorite drink is gin and tonic, and since I travel so much, I typically drank a lot of them. I decided as I started my weight-loss journey that after the first drink, I would start ordering sparkling water with lime. It looks just like a gin and tonic and is just as refreshing!"

CHAPTER 15

Being Unstoppable

In our coaching experiences, we have heard lists of excuses, ranging from irrational to comical, for why losing weight and keeping it off is impossible. It's amazing how creative people can be when it comes to justifying why they can't eat healthier and move more.

One client shared that she was unable to eat many healthy foods because of food allergies and that this is why she had been unsuccessful thus far at losing weight. When pressed for specifics, it turned out that she was only allergic to three foods: avocados, almond skins, and melons. We pointed out that eliminating those choices did not significantly limit her healthy food options and offered many other suggestions, including a list of fruits and vegetables that she *could* eat. But she dismissed these ideas, saying that she was a "picky eater" and knew she would never eat those kinds of foods. Instead of working to expand the variety of healthy foods in her diet and change her tastes, she was hiding behind her food allergies and her pickiness as challenges she couldn't overcome.

Along with these kinds of excuses, however, we have also heard heart-wrenching stories that illustrate the magnitude of the challenges people face in their efforts to lose weight: paths filled with burden and setback, including 60-hour work schedules, caring for sick parents, and debilitating injuries.

Your likelihood of falling victim to excuses or real life difficulties is increased by rushing headlong into your weight-loss journey. If you rely on emotions like disgust, anger, and frustration as motivation to work harder, these negative emotions ultimately will backfire and lead to an inner struggle that is counterproductive.

To overcome your excuses, real life challenges, and the undermining effects of negative emotions, you'll need to become "unstoppable." This is defined by a resilience of spirit and strong resolve: an understanding that life is an adventure and a challenge, all at the same time.

Once you gain the skills and understanding you need to truly become unstoppable, you will experience joy, gratitude, and happiness that are not based on the scale and that don't evaporate at the first sign of difficulty. Your enthusiasm will be impenetrable because you will thoroughly embrace the ups and downs of your weight-loss journey. You will make healthy food choices and seek ways to be active because these things make you feel nourished, empowered, and genuinely happy. When the going gets tough, instead of asking "what now?" and sinking into despair, you will simply ask "what's next?" and seek out new strategies to help you overcome an obstacle or new challenge.

THINKING SHIFT: PUT ACCEPTANCE FIRST

It is a common misconception that losing weight will lead to greater self-acceptance. In our experience, weight loss is more often a result of acceptance than the other way around. Instead of waiting until you reach your goal weight to see the positives in your life, look for them now, be grateful for what you have, and watch how the door to change opens up.

Be a Positive Voice for Change

We have encountered many clients who rely on chastising or even degrading themselves as motivation to lose weight. They believe that they can force personal action through embarrassment or shame.

There is a scene in *An Officer and a Gentleman* where Louis Gossett Jr.'s drill sergeant character, Foley, is berating recruit Zack Mayo, played by Richard Gere, by spraying him with a hose and yelling obscenities. Foley is trying to "make or break" Mayo by bringing him to his knees. In the movie, that motivational tactic worked because Mayo had a lot to prove and nothing else to turn to. This leads to one of the most famous lines from the movie: Mayo yells at Foley, "I got nowhere else to go!"

You, on the other hand, *do* have places to go. You can quit your diet. You can stop going to the gym. Other plans, other options will come along. You don't have to put up with the drill sergeant's rant; you can simply walk away. Because you can, and will, walk away from incessant criticism, negative self-talk is one of the most powerful obstacles to maintaining healthy lifestyle choices. This connection is easier to see if you imagine someone at your gym diminishing every effort you make and shaming you for the way you look. If that were actually happening, you would quit going. But it's no different when your own inner voice is the one being negative. In fact, negative self-talk is an even more powerful obstacle because it is insidious. By telling yourself you're not worth it, you're getting nowhere, or you're ugly or uncoordinated, you can talk yourself out of following your plan without even knowing that you're doing it. Without sharpening your awareness to better "hear" and contradict negative self-talk, its sabotaging impact will go unnoticed until one day you simply won't have the motivation to continue.

Positive self-talk is what truly opens the door for change to occur. If you don't appreciate all that you have going for you and believe that you're capable of change or worthy of the rewards that come with it, you'll never achieve it.

Think back to a time when maybe a parent, boss, or coach "let you have it" in an effort to get you back on track. Chances are that if it worked, if it really motivated you, then whoever was letting you have it probably did so by focusing on the issue at hand—your behavior or performance— and not on you as a person. Tough love is still love. When a great sports coach comes down hard on a player, it's a way of reminding that player to dig deeper and do what she is capable of doing. When a tough but respectful mother demands more of a child's effort in school, it's because she believes in the child's ability and wants to foster a good work ethic. The pressure and the expectations are high, but they are backed up by lots of praise, support, and caring. Neither the athlete nor the child doubts his or her value as a person.

It turns out that it is not only possible to love yourself and work to improve yourself at the same time, but that the healthy self-esteem that comes from that love is actually *necessary* to effect change. By being a positive and encouraging—instead of negative and degrading— coach for yourself, you can lay the foundation for real and lasting weight-loss success.

Value and Honor Your Body

We often hear clients express shame or disgust about their bodies. Many feel as though their bodies are working against them: It seems that they can gain weight by "just looking at a piece of cake," and they don't see any results "no matter what they do." We are dedicated to helping our clients appreciate the power and beauty of their bodies because this self-confidence is key to maintaining the motivation to eat healthy and exercise and to creating a positive and even enjoyable cycle of change. You don't need the strength or musculature of an Olympic athlete to go dancing, take a stroll on the beach, or play with your kids. Even seemingly sedentary pursuits require us to be physical in some ways, such as sightseeing or going to the theatre. This is quite a revelation to those people who have no desire to become an athlete and have not, up until now, seen any point in exercise.

For those of you who do revel in the physical aspects of this journey, there are ample rewards. You will get fit enough to hike in the mountains, take a karate class, learn to kayak, or compete in a 10-K or triathlon. Appreciate what your body can do and how it can adapt to the challenges you give it. In return, it will take you where you want to go.

Pursue Happiness

You have probably seen the bumper stickers that say, "Don't postpone joy." This is a very fitting assertion for our culture, where so many people put off happiness for later, when they believe they'll have more money, meet someone special, or weigh less than they do now. It may seem crazy to you

---

The Connection of the Intellectual and the Physical

One individual we worked with said that she loved to go to art museums, but since gaining a lot of weight, she didn't have the confidence that she could go and be able to stand and soak in the wonderful art. "I've lived my life as an intellectual, not a physical person," she said. "But what I now realize, as my physical abilities disappear in front of my eyes, is that I cannot live life as a 'floating head.' To do the things I truly enjoy, I have to get to them. My body gives me access to those things, and I need to treat it like the friend it is."

that it's okay to be happy *before* the scale shows you that ultimate number. You may believe that losing weight is the key to improving all of the aspects of your life with which you are dissatisfied. But the opposite is true.

When you stop putting off everything that brings you joy until after you lose the weight, the stress of how long it could take to reach your goal weight is diminished or eliminated. You're better able to experience the pleasure in your journey and be grateful for the victories and rewards along the way: starting or strengthening relationships, finding a new job, going back to school, and having an exciting social life.

Rather than waiting until the scale gives you permission to be happy, we encourage you to use your desire to get more out of life as the catalyst of change. We are pleasure-seeking creatures, so let your path be determined by your desires, not your regrets or fears. If you believe that you are worthy of being happy now, you will create a space for positive energy to grow. You'll seek out ways to be happier, such as by sharing your feelings with a friend, instead of just covering up your emotions with food. You'll seek out ways to use your energy and fitness for fun and pleasure, such as by going for a long walk, instead of just downing a cup of coffee.

Note: Many people rely on extra weight to protect themselves from feelings of disappointment, anger, or regret about a relationship. You can blame the lack of desire for or satisfaction with relationships on your weight and not have to take action to meet someone, to make a relationship better, or to end it. In this way, weight becomes a shield; it's a comfort to you. If this is true for you, the advice and exercises in *Coach Yourself Thin* might be helpful. But for issues that are resistant to coaching yourself, we recommend that you seek help from a certified wellness coach or, in cases of deeper issues related to body image and relationships, work with a trained behavioral counselor. (See the Resources on page 273.)

"A-Ha" Exercise

Describing a Friend Exercise: Imagine that a friend of yours wants you to describe his or her looks in detail. It's essential that your description be accurate and as thorough as possible. You can choose any words you like, but you cannot lie to protect your friend's feelings. The catch is that your friend looks exactly like you. How would you go about being accurate and honest and yet gentle and caring? In what areas would you be most gentle or supportive? What positive areas would you emphasize? How does the

I'm Coaching Myself Thin!
PUT ACCEPTANCE FIRST

Ryan: "I have developed three very positive views:

1. I'm not worthless. People like me and I have a lot of good to offer the world.

2. There is so much I want to do that I gave up on a long time ago and now it's all possible.

3. I can do things now that I could never do as a kid. I'm strong, both physically and mentally, and that's important. My attitude toward myself and the world is more positive than it has ever been before and I like the way that feels."

Renee: "Losing weight doesn't create happiness or self-acceptance in and of itself. But on the flip side, self-acceptance can indeed bring about happiness and make losing a whole lot easier! Once I was able to accept myself for who I am NOW and realize my worth is in no way tied to the number that shows up on the scale, I felt a sense of joy I can hardly describe AND a sureness about being able to continue this lifestyle for good that I'd never before experienced. This was the toughest for me to get a handle on, but the most rewarding."

language you use with your friend when being gentle and positive differ from the language you might normally use with yourself?

The next time you're inclined to criticize yourself, remember the letter you wrote to your "friend" and use the same type of words and tactics that you used there. How does this shift affect how you feel?

THINKING SHIFT: TAKE BACK CONTROL

Diets are meant to be broken, but a "lifestyle" is just what the name implies: It's for a lifetime. This is an important concept to grasp when it comes to weight loss because while you may be able to imagine following a restrictive plan for a few weeks or months, it's much harder to see yourself following any "plan" for the rest of your life. At some point, it must simply become what you do and how you live.

When you are able to see this larger picture, you will realize that no one decision is a deal breaker; no single missed meal or unplanned indulgence or missed exercise session can knock you off track. Success becomes something you measure by consistency over the long-term, not perfection over the short-term.

It might sound paradoxical, then, to recommend that you "live in the moment" after we've painted the big picture as being so important. But living in the moment and keeping the big picture in mind aren't mutually exclusive. It works like "Think globally, act locally," a philosophy that has been used in various contexts, including city planning, environmental action, and business strategy.

"Think globally" means understanding how your actions affect the whole planet. Big-picture thinking, when it comes to weight loss, can help you realize that it's all of your behaviors, not just your most recent meal, that affects your weight and your health.

"Act locally" means making changes where you have the most control: That means changing yourself, your home, and your community. It's all well and good to want to make the planet a better place, but if you just sat at home and worried about how you could possibly influence world peace

Big Picture Thinking and the Scale

Have you ever eaten a meal or exercised and then weighed yourself immediately afterward, either lamenting your "gain" or celebrating your "loss"? Don't put too much stock in an individual reading on the scale, because when it comes to weigh-ins, big-picture thinking is a must. Any weight gain or loss that occurs over the course of a meal or an exercise session, or even within a few hours of either, is due mostly to fluctuations in the amounts of food and liquid in your body. These gains and losses are not permanent.

A weekly weigh-in, on the other hand, is more likely to give you an accurate picture of what is going on, although it too may be skewed by water retention following a higher sodium meal or a heavy exercise session. You'll get a better indication of whether or not your plan is working by comparing your weigh-ins over the course of several weeks.

or hunger, you'd probably never do much about it. By finding a local way to make changes, you're more likely and better equipped to actually take action. Likewise, when you're trying to lose weight, it can be intimidating to look at everything you have to change and how far you have to go to reach your goals. It can paralyze you into not changing anything at all. By living in the moment, you can focus just on what you can do today to bring about those changes. If you want to eat more fruits and vegetables, you can start with your next snack or meal. If you've missed a couple of exercise sessions, take a look at your day planner and find your next opportunity. You're living in the moment, focusing on the daily healthy behaviors that add up to a healthy life, but you're never losing sight of the big picture and the understanding that it is consistency and not perfection with those behaviors that is the key to success.

Use Permission and Forgiveness

Once you make your break from small-picture "diet" thinking, you will begin to see your eating and exercise habits against the backdrop of the rest of your life. It is true that we all have to navigate a world full of stress and distraction that is poorly suited to a healthy lifestyle, so thank goodness being perfect is not required for long-term success. That would leave most of us without much hope of ever making lasting change! But if you are not expected to be perfect, how will you ever make progress? If you constantly let yourself off the hook, how will you lose weight?

Not aiming for perfection doesn't mean that you don't aim for solid, challenging goals: It just means being more flexible. Aim to keep your calorie intake within a range, instead of at an exact level; exercise 4 to 6 days each week instead of every day; and allow yourself a splurge or a rest day occasionally. Remember when we discussed the concept of 80/20 living on page 66? Living an 80/20 lifestyle requires that you give yourself real permission—permission without negative self-talk or guilt attached—to be less than perfect. That way, one slip does not slingshot you from being a motivated go-getter to a couch potato. You are conscious of your choice and the reasons you're making it—a celebration, the need for a break—and you are able to tell the difference between being flexible and being off track.

When you do go off track, you need to be able to recognize it and, without judging or berating yourself, get right back in sync with your

I'm Coaching Myself Thin!
TAKE BACK CONTROL

Ryan: "I always used to find some excuse to blame society, my parents, the school system, the media; but none of those people forced me to eat the way I did and not exercise. It's just very freeing to know now that nobody is controlling my life but me. I accept my faults, mistakes, and slips and move on. I have changed the way I think about myself and realize that I am worth it, even when I mess up."

Jen: "When I realized that I controlled my own choices, it really did change things for me. I realized I didn't have to eat the things everyone else ate, even if they tried to push the food on me. It was *my* decision. It also became clear that my emotions didn't have to dictate what I ate. Taking back control takes the power away from the guilt and makes it easier to forgive yourself."

goals. To bounce back quickly, you will need the power of forgiveness. Dwelling on the slip, wallowing in self-blame, or passing the responsibility for your choices onto other people or circumstances only deepens the hole you've begun to dig for yourself. Forgiveness provides the ladder to climb out and move on.

The Choice Is Yours

There is incredible power in making your own choices. You're free from the constraints of someone else's idea of how you should live healthy and lose weight. This independence sweeps away the victim mentality. It's no longer society's fault that you can't find healthy food in a restaurant, your boss's responsibility that you can't eat healthy on the job, or your spouse's attitude that keeps you from exercise.

What stops many people from appreciating the power to choose is that with this power comes personal responsibility for the results of those choices. Taking control of your choices and accepting responsibility for their outcomes requires shifting from an external to an internal locus of control.

With an external locus of control, you tend to attribute what happens to you to things beyond your control; you blame other people, aspects of your personality or skills that you believe you cannot change, or just plain luck. If you come up short on a project at work, you might say, "You never told me how to use that program. It's not my fault I didn't get my work done," or "Dang, I can't do this. I'm way too lazy to learn how to use that program."

In the face of astounding success, you might say, "Wow, what luck. I can't believe that idea actually worked. The customer must not have spotted all of my mistakes."

With an internal locus of control, however, you focus on what is within your control and take responsibility for your own decisions and actions. Revisiting the workplace scenario, if you don't meet expectations, you might say, "My skills just weren't as sharp as they needed to be, but I'll be ready next time," or "I'll come up with a better plan for managing my work time in the future." If you set a company record for sales, you would believe that it was because of your skill as a salesperson and accept the honor graciously.

As long as you relinquish control of your choices and responsibility for the results to something or someone else, you will only succeed when the circumstances are exactly right. When you take back your power to choose your path and accept credit for the outcomes, you give yourself the opportunity for lasting success.

"A-Ha" Exercise

Big Picture Exercise: Find two clear jars or containers. Count out 365 pennies—one for each day of the year—and pour them into one of the jars or containers. Take a penny out and put it into the empty jar for each day of the coming year that you anticipate not being able to meet your nutrition and exercise goals as you would like. Make sure you account for holidays that are special to you, your vacations, as well as birthdays and special gatherings. If you have a stressful time of the year at work, put pennies in for those days.

When you have thought of every day that you believe you will be unable to stick with your lifestyle goals, what do the jars look like?

Look at the jar that started out as "perfection" and imagine each coin as a day when you will have the opportunity to make healthy choices. Compare it to the other jar, and look at those coins as the days when it will be more difficult to make healthy choices.

How does the comparison make you feel? Does it seem more possible for you to lose weight by breaking free of All-or-Nothing Thinking and focusing on the days where you do have more control?

This exercise does not suggest that you have no control over your choices during vacations, holidays, special gatherings, or stressful times at work. Rather, it opens your eyes to the idea that you can make progress by focusing on the days when control is easier for you. It is possible to enjoy days that take you away from your normal routine, such as a day off from exercise or the chance to have a favorite dessert, without going off the deep end and giving up on your plan entirely.

THINKING SHIFT: BE RESILIENT

There is a chance that even if you work diligently on making your environment a supportive one, it may present challenges that defy your best planning and efforts to remain flexible. When this happens, you'll need to be resilient to be successful.

Stand Your Ground

Being resilient means that you are not swayed by someone else's opinion of you, your abilities, or your chances of success. Someone else does not decide your future. You may discover that many of the opinions and criticisms that influence you come from casual acquaintances or total strangers—people that don't have much influence over your day-to-day life. How much control do you want to hand over to people who don't know you well, if at all, and who certainly don't care about you?

If you want to walk in your local park or work out at the gym, let that decision be your own. If someone is hateful enough to make a contemptuous comment, stay focused on what you can control. While you can't change his words, you can change your reaction to them. By viewing his negativity as something brought on by his anger and ill will toward others in general, rather than you specifically, you are able to put it into its proper place. Letting his unkindness roll off of you limits his influence over you to mere seconds, and he has no more impact on your well-being than a rude driver on the highway would.

It is also possible that what you perceive to be a condescending look is nothing at all, or that a person you think is laughing at you hasn't even noticed you. We have all been in situations where we wondered, "Are they making fun of me?" only to find out that our fears were unfounded.

Resilience is a skill that must be cultivated. The Quick Fix Mentality has overridden our ability to persist in the face of obstacles and difficulty. It has become commonplace to seek convenience and ease.

The difference between those who make healthy changes successfully and those who don't is not a lack of setbacks, but the ability to get back on track quickly. To make changes that stick, it takes a bit of good old elbow grease and stubbornness.

Dare to Be Different

We have discussed the effort it takes to swim against the current of modern society. In order to stick with the changes you make, you'll also need to be able to tolerate the feeling of being, well, a little different. As we mentioned in Creating Successful Environments, you will probably encounter sideways glances or little rolls of the eyes. And the thought might creep into your head that, maybe, this business of being healthy is starting to wear a little thin.

We've been conditioned to believe that our health should only be a high priority when we're sick. It's common and acceptable to take medicine to combat illness, but it's downright strange to refuse to eat in a restaurant that doesn't offer healthy options or stay in a hotel that doesn't have an adequate gym. Chances are, you'll encounter many situations that draw attention to the fact that you don't "fit in"—family gatherings, business and social events, and vacations and holidays, to name a few. You'll encounter people who don't understand why you exercise or why you eat the way you do. They'll marvel that you walk or run distances they would only tackle in a car, and they'll question you about what diet you're on, how much weight you've lost, and how long it'll be before you can eat "normally" again.

You'll have to tactfully turn down unhealthy food that is constantly pushed in your direction, ask to go to or *not* go to particular restaurants, or bring food into restaurants to supplement what you are able to order off the menu. To fit in exercise, you'll have to constantly schedule it into your plans for the day and protect that time as if it's just another meeting.

You'll also encounter frustrated dieters who want your company. When you stubbornly refuse to buy into their latest fad, they will smirk. And when you continue to ask for a side of steamed veggies instead of indulging in French fries, they will goad you to give in. They'll tell you that "just one cookie" or "one little weekend off your exercise plan" won't hurt.

Revel in being different and let society catch up. Eventually your family, friends, and co-workers will realize that the changes you've made are for good. And eventually you won't feel as self-conscious doing something or asking for something that helps you stay healthy.

Celebrate Your Victories, Focus on Your Strengths

It's no secret that doing well makes you feel good—euphoric, even—and one of the keys to being resilient is learning how to tap into this feeling when things don't seem to be going your way. It may take a bit of looking, but finding the positive during tough times can be enough to carry you through until you're back on your feet.

Ask yourself the following:

What is going well with my healthy eating and/or exercise?

What am I enjoying about being healthier?

What did I do well today?

Now finish these statements:

Because I'm healthier and more fit, I'm looking forward to_____.

I'm happy about_____.

I'm thankful for_____.

Your responses are important windows into the areas of your life from which you can draw positive energy. Recognizing your nonscale victories (NSVs; see page 52) reminds you of the richness you add to your life by being healthy and active. These NSVs can help put you back on track when you feel as though you've lost your drive and focus.

These everyday victories also give you ample chances to reward yourself for a job well done. A tangible reward like a new pair of jeans, a massage, or even a weekend away can make all the difference when it comes to maintaining your inner fire.

When you do get off track, focus on your own personal skills and strengths to help pull you back. We are all blessed with particular gifts.

I'm Coaching Myself Thin!

BE RESILIENT

Renee: "Now I realize that one bad choice is just one bad choice. I can still make my next choice a good one. I don't even think of it as falling off the wagon anymore. It used to be: 'Okay, I'm off track—let's grab everything we can.' Now it doesn't control me like that. Realizing this made me stop and think about all of my past slips (and the frustrations of the recovery that come with it) in a different light. This year I discovered that I do have the ability to get through, with my health intact. I can see that my confidence has grown with time and likely as a result of what I've made it through thus far."

Tricia: Tricia discovered the power of daring to be different. She stood up for her lifestyle until others in her life thought of her in a whole new way. "I remember when my sister first began to identify me as an 'exerciser.' I was visiting her, and we had plans to go shopping the next day. Before bed, she said, 'And of course you will have to get in your walk in the morning. So, as soon as you're back, we'll have some breakfast and we'll be off!' I was floored by this recognition and by the magnitude of what it meant to be seen in this light. How cool to not have to ask for that time. She just *knew*."

Maybe you have a lot of courage and a strong sense of adventure: You've started your own business, traveled extensively, or gone back to school after years in the workforce. Lean on those strengths and try out a new exercise class, recipe, or ethnic food.

Perhaps you are a social person who thrives on teamwork or in a group. It comes naturally for you to organize your book club or schedule outings for your golf foursome. Use that talent to start a walking group or cooking club or to recruit friends to sign up for group personal training at your local gym.

"A-Ha" Exercise

Resilience Exercise: Here is a terrific metaphor developed by Judy Wilson, owner of Team iRun in Knoxville, Tennessee, and Lori Shepard, USATF Level I instructor, to describe how people react differently to adversity and/or negative feedback. People can be described as:

Walnuts: They're tough and resilient and can bounce back from adversity; they're able to resist other people's doubts and criticisms.

Apples: These people put up a positive front but bruise on the inside, which eventually tears them down from the inside out.

Eggs: This group is overly susceptible to criticism and doubt; they have fragile self-esteem and shaky confidence.

Track your emotional reactions for a day. When faced with adversity, negative outcomes, or criticism, are you mostly a walnut, an apple, or an egg?

Are there certain people, environments, or situations that make you more susceptible to being an apple or an egg?

What can you do to be more resilient around people who would bruise or crack you? Brainstorm about your personal strengths. Take 5 minutes to write down as many as you can think of. Review your list and circle any that you feel would be useful for being more resilient when facing the people, environments, or situations that make you feel most vulnerable.

CHAPTER 16

Awakening Your Intuition

Imagine waking in the middle of the night to the scream of your smoke alarm. You get out of bed, but instead of looking around for fire or any signs of smoke, you pull the smoke alarm down from the ceiling, remove the batteries, and go back to sleep. That would be a very risky move. Similarly, people today often try to suppress and ignore what their bodies are telling them so they don't have to take the time or energy to truly assess what is going on.

The Quick Fix Mindset would have you believe that even though you are experiencing headaches, sore joints, heartburn, insomnia, or even depression, you don't need to change your behavior. Rather, you should override any discomfort with a painkiller, neutralize your heartburn with an antacid, zap your insomnia with a few sleeping pills, and boost your mood with an antidepressant. While these medications are effective at keeping you moving forward and managing your discomfort, taking them routinely is like taking the batteries out of the smoke alarm: You have not put out the fire, and you're leaving yourself in harm's way. You are not changing any behaviors to address the underlying problems. Instead, you are silencing what your body is telling you because it isn't what you want to hear.

What might happen if you completely changed your reaction from numbing out to active listening, where you invite better communication and begin working *with* your body, thoughts, and emotions? If you are tired of "managing" all of your symptoms, awakening is exactly what you need, and it very well may be the piece that's been missing from your weight-loss puzzle.

THINKING SHIFT: TUNE IN TO YOUR BODY

What may be driving your food choices more than anything else at this moment is what tastes good and what satisfies your appetite, even if it's an artificial food. Tuning in to your body involves distinguishing what you *want* from what your body *needs* for optimal functioning. You may not enjoy drinking water, for instance, but if you remind yourself that your body needs water to produce energy, and then factor in that you want to feel better and perform better, you will find that water is suddenly much more appealing!

The next time you question whether you should eat a particular food, imagine that your taste buds are turned off. Would you still eat it? If you were eating more to satisfy your hunger and not just for pleasure or comfort, you would find it easy to eat salmon, broccoli, and brown rice. It's just the same as putting quality gasoline in your car for the sake of your car's performance.

But isn't eating supposed to be pleasurable? Definitely—but there is a balance between eating for pleasure and eating to nourish your body. Another shift in your thinking, and one that you may find hard to believe at the moment, is that the healthier you become, the more you will enjoy eating healthier food.

Taste

If our goal in America is to make rich-tasting food, then we're doing an amazing job. Restaurants and food manufacturers have perfected recipes that satisfy your cravings for salt, sugar, and fat. Unfortunately, with this trifecta of temptations at your fingertips, following your taste buds can be hazardous to your health.

How your taste buds work is encoded in your genetics, and these genes haven't changed much in the last 40,000 years. Back then, eating to satisfy your desire for sweet, oily, and salty foods worked wonders for your health because foods with these flavors—like berries, seeds, and sea vegetables— were packed with vital nutrients. But in more recent years, we've figured out ways to concentrate these flavors and blend them into processed foods that are stripped of essential nutrients.

Tuning in to your preferred tastes will help you identify your "trigger" foods, or those that you struggle to eat in moderation. By recognizing the tastes and textures that you find tempting—salty and crunchy, like potato chips; sweet, like cookies; or creamy, like ice cream—you can see temptation coming and head it off before it strikes. And this heightened awareness will also help you identify healthier versions of these tastes and textures and incorporate them into your program as treats.

	PREHISTORIC DAYS	MODERN DAY
Sweet	Berries and tree fruits	Soft drinks, baked goods, and candy
Salty	Seafood and root vegetables	Hamburgers, pizza, and chips
Oily	Nuts, seeds, and coconut	French fries and salad dressings

As a result of eating a "cleaner" diet (see Chapter 17, starting on page 116), your taste buds will become more sensitized to sugar, salt, and oil. What tasted delicious to you before may soon taste too salty, too sweet, or too oily. This kind of feedback from your body helps you steer clear of many of your less-healthy restaurant or fast-food favorites.

Hunger

In a culture of oversize portions, habitual eating, and absentminded grazing, it's no surprise that you are not clear on your hunger and fullness signals. Did you finish that mound of pasta because you were hungry or because it was there in front of you? Did you buy that muffin because you were hungry or because you wanted something sweet to nibble on while you rode the subway? And where the heck did that whole sleeve of cookies go while you were watching TV?

Believe it or not, in our diet-crazed culture, undereating and skipping meals contribute just as much to our eating woes as overindulging does. Think of how a pendulum swings from one side to the other; if you undereat, the hunger builds and your blood sugar level drops, setting you up to overeat in the afternoon or evening, when the pendulum has swung to the other side. The goal is to find a balance where you are never overly hungry or overly full.

You will benefit more by keeping tabs on your hunger than by trying to ignore or suppress it. As you bring your awareness to your hunger signals throughout the day (see Hunger and Fullness Scale on page 135), you will begin to recognize when you are physically hungry, rather than having an emotional craving due to stress, boredom, or being upset. You'll understand when you need to have a snack, and you'll learn to stop eating before you are too full. Being more aware of your hunger signals can also help you tune in to which foods are more filling relative to their calorie count, such as fruit, salads, and cooked vegetables.

Hydration Status

Your body is made up of roughly 60 percent water, and it's very easy to become dehydrated. Take steps to stay adequately hydrated by following the guidelines for proper hydration on page 121. On the other hand, it's also surprisingly common for your body to retain excess water when it's recovering from a hard workout; after a high-sodium meal or snack; during your menstrual cycle (if you're a woman); or because of sickness, certain medications, and air travel.

When you step on the scale, it can't tell whether you are retaining water. You may have had a great week in terms of meeting your nutrition and exercise goals and have actually lost 2 pounds of body fat, but for one reason or another, your body is retaining 48 ounces of water. Those 48 ounces skew the scale 3 pounds heavier, making you think you gained a pound that week!

Remind yourself *before* you step on the scale that water weight may give you a false reading. Before you get near the scale, take a moment to reflect on your weekly goals and practice giving yourself a rating based on this reflection. Aside from monitoring your sodium intake, there's often nothing you can do about water retention except continue to exercise, choose healthy foods to help restore water balance, and be patient. Stay consistent with your water intake to facilitate normalcy, and

If you are not convinced that water can skew a single reading so significantly, try the following exercise: Weigh yourself one morning on a digital scale, then step off and drink 32 ounces of water over the course of the next 15 minutes. Step back on the scale and see how much weight you've "gained."

remember that not only is drinking enough water vital for good health and proper metabolism, staying hydrated will also help you feel better and lose weight.

Pain

In a culture that espouses the "No pain, no gain" philosophy, it is no wonder that you feel like you should push through pain if you want to get in shape and lose weight. The Quick Fix Mindset urges you to take the painkiller without even considering making lifestyle changes. It doesn't tell you that silencing the pain is like taking the batteries out of the smoke alarm, as we discussed on page 97, or that if you aren't careful, the underlying "fire" can become a torn meniscus in your knee or damage to the ligaments in your shoulder.

A healthier path is inviting communication from your body and taking steps to work with it. If your pain is not severe or debilitating, what actions can you take to slowly eliminate an indigestion medication or an over-the-counter anti-inflammatory? How many of the symptoms that you're experiencing are caused by an inflammatory diet, lack of movement, inadequate strength or flexibility, sleep deprivation, or stress? If you are in severe pain or have a more serious medical condition and eliminating medications is not an option, how much can you lessen your pain or other symptoms, and at least reduce the dosage of the medications you are taking, by changing lifestyle factors?

Experiencing pain while exercising is very different from feeling discomfort after a hard effort or the muscular soreness that sometimes follows a tough workout. Pain tells you what areas of your body are compromised and out of balance, while discomfort from effort and soreness are both normal results of exercise. In the course of improving your fitness level and becoming stronger and more physically fit, you will likely experience discomfort and occasional soreness. (We'll cover how to tell the difference between pain, discomfort, and soreness in Part 5.)

Energy

If you reach for coffee, soda, or an energy drink as a daily "pick me up," that's a pretty clear sign that you are suffering from an energy shortage. Perhaps you don't believe that healthy foods and physical activity could

I'm Coaching Myself Thin!
TUNE IN TO YOUR BODY

Tricia: Trish used to be a pro at eating on autopilot. "I thought I needed a soda every afternoon to ward off a headache, a fancy latte most mornings on the way to work, and a homemade chai and biscotti for an evening treat," she says. Trish realized that she didn't like this mindless relationship she was having with food. She began listening to her body and thinking about how much more satisfied she felt after she ate an apple and some almonds in place of that soda, or how a short walk in the evening gave her way more energy than dessert. "My schedule is so busy, but I can either allow the circumstances of my life to dictate my choices, or I can use my choices to dictate how I face the circumstances of my life," she says.

Steven: "I've had a number of injuries on this journey. Historically, I would have just given up when I felt the pain, but now I know that I just need to take a step back and replan. I pay attention now more than ever and don't push my luck. One serious injury that happened because I didn't listen to my body could have a major long-term impact."

ever give you the same feeling, but you've never been able to quit these "crutches" for long enough to find out.

One of the keys to having more energy is increasing your energy production. Behaviors that help you produce more energy include consuming the right amount of nutrient-dense food, consistently getting moderate exercise, drinking enough water, and getting enough quality sleep. Note that with each of these factors, balance is essential: Proper calorie intake for your size and activity level leaves you feeling energized while overeating causes you to feel lethargic. The appropriate amount of exercise for your fitness level can send your energy levels soaring to new heights, but if you overdo it, you will feel more tired and irritable than invigorated. Drinking enough water for your body (see the guidelines for proper hydration on page 121) and for the climate you live in prevents dehydration and increases your work capacity, but too much is not better. (Overconsuming water in a short period of time can make you very ill.) And the same goes for sleep; it's the key to feeling energized, but too much can lead to sluggishness.

It's also essential to conserve your energy throughout the day, so be aware of your main energy drains. Common ones include too much stress, caffeine, refined sugar, fast food, alcohol, certain medications, and inadequate sleep. Think about what you can change to better preserve your energy for the things you need and want to do.

Waking up to and fully experiencing your body's physical sensations will help you make informed decisions about what your body needs and what does and does not work for you when it comes to food choices and exercise. As you become more aware, you'll be much better equipped to coach yourself through the challenges of lifestyle change.

"A-Ha" Exercise

Note: Jon Kabat-Zinn, PhD, developed the mindfulness-based stress reduction program and uses raisins as a teaching tool for increasing self-awareness. This exercise is adapted from his work.[1]

Mindful Raisin Exercise: Allow yourself 10 minutes for this exercise. With a single raisin in hand, find a quiet spot where you can close your eyes and relax. Take a deep breath and begin imagining where your raisin came from: See the beautifully kept vineyard under a bright blue sky; picture the field of luscious grapevines. Envision freshly harvested grapes drying on the ground beside the vines. One of those dried grapes is now in your hand. Slowly smell your raisin, paying close attention to the subtle aromas. Next, place the raisin in your mouth and let it sit on your tongue. Roll it around and notice how it feels. Tune in to everything that you can taste and smell in the moment. Savor it. Slowly bite the raisin and notice the intensity of the flavor it releases.

Over the next minute or two, see how much you can taste this raisin. And when you're ready, go ahead and swallow it.

How was this raisin different than others you've eaten? Take a few minutes of reflection and write down your observations.

As you eat your meals over the next month, use the savoring skills you practiced in the Mindful Raisin Exercise. As you slow down and consider the flavors and textures, notice the ways it changes your enjoyment of the foods on your plate.

THINKING SHIFT: TUNE IN TO YOUR MIND

You have thousands of thoughts racing through your mind each day. All of us do. Many of these thoughts are fleeting and have no bearing on your life, while others are more daunting, like thinking that you will never reach your weight-loss goal because of how far you have to go. You may replay these thoughts often enough that, even if they are not accurate, you begin to believe that they are the truth. Your mind is a powerful tool, and what you imagine to be often comes true, whether that thing is negative or positive. For example, you may not view yourself as a good public speaker, so before a presentation at work you begin to think about how you will blow it. And, lo and behold, when your time comes to speak you stutter and stumble and totally embarrass yourself.

On the flip side of the coin, what would happen if you thought about being capable of navigating a dinner party and being able to stick to healthy food choices? Chances are, if you envision ways to succeed before you enter a situation, you will be much more successful when the moment arrives.

Tuning in to how you think throughout the day is essential to successfully coaching yourself through lifestyle changes. It's the first step in turning your thoughts from barriers to assets. You can replace negative thoughts with empowered and positive thoughts that steer you in the direction that you want to go.

Thoughts and Judgment

Awareness of your thoughts allows you to see where judgment comes into play and recognize the impact that those judgments have on your success. Many of your thoughts do have a judgmental quality, which is often essential for your well-being; those thoughts guide you to make important decisions that protect your safety and your health. For example, it is often necessary to judge whether it's safe to walk to your car alone, or you may judge correctly that a co-worker is out to sabotage your diet and decide to keep up your guard around her.

However, when you negatively judge yourself, your body, and your ability to stick with your weight-loss program, you undermine yourself and plant the seeds of failure.

Thoughts and Emotions

Thoughts are often tinged with emotions, both negative and positive. Sometimes these will surface based on past experiences. If you think for a few moments about a humiliating experience you had earlier in life, you may feel awkward and ashamed. Think of a cherished memory, though, and you might feel proud or excited. Even though there is nothing "real" about the old experience in your present moment, your brain links the memory with strong emotions and the thought of it brings those feelings back up. And if you're thrust into a situation that brings up that memory, the emotions will come rushing back, as well.

It is possible to release the emotions associated with a negative experience. Time and distance may help you distill the memory and see that there is no reason to be controlled by it today. Relinquishing control over the incident can help: As you come to realize that you can't change it, you may also realize that you don't have to. You can go forward without having to prove anything to those involved or even resolve anything. Understanding that your past does not have to be your current truth is a powerful step.

You can actively create positive thoughts and emotions about a situation as well. For instance, as you approach the dinner party in the example above, you can imagine replacing appetizers with just a glass of wine, or even a club soda with a splash of cranberry juice and a cherry. Picture yourself drinking that and having a great time, and your confidence grows by leaps and bounds *before* you arrive at the party.

Emotional Eating

When people succumb to emotional eating and reach for so-called "comfort foods," it is usually a way of self-medicating and covering up feelings. Tuning in to your mind gives you the ability to manage your urges to eat or drink for emotional reasons. Without mental awareness, emotional eating is a knee-jerk reaction: The feelings of discomfort automatically lead to eating. With mental awareness, you create an opportunity to ask yourself some important questions regarding the connection between your emotions and your eating choices. If you're contending with the urge to eat, follow this series of questions and responses.

- Ask, "Am I physically hungry right now?" If the answer is yes, eat something healthy; you're done with the quiz. If the answer is no, go to question 2.

- Ask, "What am I feeling right now?" If possible, label the emotion you're feeling and who or what is causing it.

- Ask, "What do I *need* right now?" Look back at your answer to question 2. Depending on the emotion you are experiencing, you may feel that it could help to journal about it, talk to a friend about it, or do something nice for yourself that is unrelated to food.

In Part 6, we will outline in more detail some strategies and skills that will help you navigate those times when emotions are threatening to knock your healthy behaviors off track.

Experience Your Emotions

Earlier in this chapter we discussed the trap of judging yourself too harshly. A similar trap is judging yourself for the feelings and emotions that you have instead of giving yourself "space" to feel what you are feeling. A humiliating experience may stir up strong emotions, but if you jump to judging these emotions, you will make the experience even more painful.

Keep in mind that it is not only negative emotions that trigger this response. Many people are unable to fully receive good fortune and will also squash emotions they deem to be "too" positive. When things go right in their lives and they have every reason to be happy, they feel guilty for their good luck or fretful that the happiness will soon come to an end, and they try to suppress the positive feelings.

If emotional eating is an issue for you, a big part of the problem could actually be physical. Be sure that you're doing the following:

- Getting enough sleep.
- Engaging in regular exercise.
- Keeping healthy food on hand and readily available.
- Keeping the tempting junk out of sight as much as possible.
- Establishing a consistent eating plan.

I'm Coaching Myself Thin!

TUNE IN TO YOUR MIND

Renee: "I always used to think I just ate from stress, but I've come to realize that I crave food when I feel emotionally empty. It could be anything from missing talking with a friend to being down about not having found someone to spend my life with. The act of recognizing that has freed me. Instances of emotional eating have diminished for me and aren't nearly as damaging as they once were when they do occur. They are short-lived and low-calorie. Now I stop in the moment and try to recognize what I am feeling. My main strategy is to notice how my body is feeling physically and to take a moment to ask myself, 'What is it that I really want or need?' I've found I can usually find the answer and when I do, it becomes apparent to me that food won't meet that particular need. That is enough to make it go away, a lot of times."

Jen: "I feel like I am more in control of the emotions than I ever have been before. I can allow myself to feel and experience the emotions (no matter how uncomfortable they make me at times) without losing control and doing or saying something that I'll later regret. And that measure of peace that is thrown in there really does help. It is a reminder to me that no matter what the emotions are right now, how painful or sad I feel, things will work out and things will be okay. I think that is what is allowing me to feel and experience the emotions without them dictating so many other things in my life . . . like eating."

You can "eat your emotions" as a short-term fix, but numbing and distracting yourself won't help you move forward. *That which you resist, persists.* Accept your struggles and doubts as normal challenges in life and allow yourself to feel positive emotions without guilt in order to succeed in your weight-loss journey. (See page 89 for more on using "real," or guilt-free, permission.)

Both positive and negative emotions help you experience a life full of richness, texture, and contrast. Deep and resonant emotions like sadness, happiness, anger, courage, frustration, and pleasure can enrich your life if you allow yourself to feel them fully. Validate your feelings instead of making yourself feel wrong for having them.

What might it look like to choose to sit with your emotions, no matter how uncomfortable, and trust that the path of healing and relief is to be with them and work through them? Maybe this is something that you cannot imagine without the support and guidance of a therapist. That's okay. But realize that you can make real headway on your own by giving yourself more space and opportunity to express your emotions, even if you are just writing in your journal or talking with a close friend.

"I am 'feeling' my feelings now instead of stuffing them down. Yeah, it kind of stinks to 'feel' them, but it is so much better than burying them. I am finding it easier and easier to talk to hubby again. The family is definitely happier with the new and improved Mom. My outlook is just so much brighter. I am starting to *like* me again. Life is good!"

—Biggest Loser Club member

Other Resources

Those who are successful with weight loss work on underlying emotional issues and develop strategies for managing emotional eating. You may be able to make significant strides by following our advice, but you may need professional help and support, as well. See the Resources on page 273 for a list of books on emotional eating; these references go beyond the scope of what is covered here. In the Resources we also provide recommendations for finding a behavioral therapist to help you access and process your thoughts and feelings.

"A-Ha" Exercise

Emotional Check-In Exercise: Over the next 24 hours, ask yourself two questions whenever you experience a strong emotion.

First question: "What am I feeling right now?"

Name the feeling. See these lists for guidance.

Examples of negative emotions:

Abandoned	Embarrassed	Sad
Afraid	Frustrated	Sorrowful
Angry	Humiliated	Undeserving
Annoyed	Ignored	Useless
Anxious	Insecure	Withdrawn
Blue	Lonely	Worried
Depressed	Melancholy	Worthless
Detached	Nervous	

Examples of positive emotions:

Amused	Enthralled	Playful
Appreciative	Excited	Proud
Cheerful	Glad	Relieved
Content	Grateful	Satisfied
Delighted	Happy	Thrilled
Eager	Hopeful	Triumphant
Ecstatic	Optimistic	
Elated	Peaceful	

Second question: "What are some strategies you can use to experience this emotion in a constructive way? Consider journaling, sharing it with a friend, diffusing it through exercise, expressing it into a painting or drawing, or soothing yourself by taking a candlelit bubble bath.

During the next month, journal about your emotions as time permits. What patterns do you notice, if any? What helps you avoid food when the urge to eat for emotional reasons surfaces? What other resources do you need to help you? (See page 273.)

THINKING SHIFT: CREATE A NEW WAY OF BEING

Awakening means opening yourself to a whole new way of being—one that may not seem possible to you at the start of your journey. Changing your way of life can help your body heal in dramatic ways by restoring balance to your cholesterol, blood pressure, and blood glucose levels. In an everyday sense, you will also notice that you will sleep better, move easier, and hurt less.

Being aware of your body's signals will help you bring balance to your eating and exercise approaches. Your taste buds change so significantly that many of your old favorites no longer taste good to you, and overeating makes you feel miserable rather than bringing you enjoyment. You notice that exercise feels good to your muscles and joints and that not moving actually increases your stiffness and fatigue. You break free of longstanding addictions to caffeine or sweets and learn to use exercise as a "pick me up" for your both your energy and your mood.. As you leave the old diet mindset behind, you learn how to enjoy a healthy balance of whole foods and controlled treats without feeling guilty. And you find that there are many forms of movement, whether a gentle walk in the park or a vigorous competition, that bring you pleasure.

The Power of Trust

If you have fallen into the trap of setting your expectations too high and then punishing yourself for coming up short, it is time to consider a brand new relationship with yourself. At the core of this new relationship is trust. You must put down the battle-ax you have wielded against yourself, learn to say yes to yourself, and believe in your ability to make better decisions. Trust means believing that your motivation is resilient and will not let you down, having confidence in the effectiveness of your plan, and knowing that you can rely on your support network to help you through.

Your ability to trust yourself is built on the foundation you created by strengthening the thinking skills in the Stepping-Stones of Part 3.

As you build trust in yourself, you will:

- Allow yourself to experience a range of healthy emotions instead of striving to dull those emotions with food.
- Take responsibility for your past actions.
- Deepen your appreciation of what your body allows you to experience daily.
- Forgive yourself for your imperfections.
- Notice your thoughts throughout the day, cherishing and celebrating the positive and choosing not to react to the negative.

- Feed yourself positive affirmations and surround yourself with supportive people.
- Listen to your hunger and fullness signals and recognize pain and exertion cues.
- Think ahead in order to manage unexpected situations.
- Ask for what you need without feeling embarrassed about taking care of yourself.

Unhealthy Lifestyle Vortex

Each choice that you make moving forward is connected to another and builds upon the one before in unimaginable ways. Perhaps you've been struggling to break free of what we call the Unhealthy Lifestyle Vortex or you're feeling stuck this very moment. If so, your life may look like this:

1. You work hard at your job and usually are too tired and stressed-out to exercise when you get home from work.

2. You don't have the time or energy to make a healthy dinner, so you stop for fast food or takeout on the way home from work, or you eat an unsatisfying frozen dinner at home.

3. Because you are stressed-out, you snack on salty or sweet foods in the evening and may have a couple of beers or other alcoholic drinks.

4. You don't sleep very well, and you may take medication to help you fall asleep.

5. You wake up feeling tired, grab a coffee, and are out the door.

6. There are temptations at work—somebody brings in cookies, another person has a jar of candy on her desk, your co-workers go out to a local buffet for lunch. You find this food hard to resist. Eating it gives you a short-term boost, but soon you find yourself riding the sugar-and-carbs roller coaster. You gain weight.

7. You are heavy and feel sluggish and depressed. You wonder if your thyroid is causing your problems. You go see your doctor, who tells you that your thyroid is fine but writes a prescription for an antidepressant to help with your mood. It helps some, but soon you notice that the medication boosts your appetite. Things get worse from here.

Healthy Lifestyle Vortex

It can be hard to escape from the Unhealthy Lifestyle Vortex, at least in the beginning. The process of getting from a stuck place to an empowered one is a journey of breaking free of the obstacles you've been facing and becoming a champion at all five Stepping-Stones: Expecting Greatness, Regaining Your Balance, Creating Successful Environments, Being Unstoppable, and Awakening Your Intuition. Imagine that you've changed your thinking, and with your new attitude you've started making changes that are helping you leap over to the Healthy Lifestyle Vortex. It looks like this:

1. You work hard at the office, but you manage your stress by taking a few breaks during the day and walking around. You practice deep breathing and make sure you are drinking enough water from the office cooler. When you get home from work, you still feel tired but decide to go to the gym anyway to work out because you know it will make you feel better.

2. After the workout, you come home and feel energized enough to make a simple, healthy dinner.

3. You still struggle with the temptation to eat after dinner, but you decide to have a cup of hot tea and read a book rather than snacking. You go to bed feeling a little better and happy that you didn't get into the cookies. (The next day you throw them away on your way to work!)

4. You sleep better, getting up only once to go to the bathroom.

5. You wake up feeling okay as you sit down for a bowl of high-fiber cereal, a sprinkling of almonds, and a piece of fruit. You make a travel mug of tea or coffee; grab a low-fat yogurt for a snack; and pack a turkey breast sandwich, baby carrots, and an apple for lunch before heading out the door.

6. There are temptations at work: Somebody brings in cookies, another person has a jar of candy on her desk, everybody goes out for pizza at lunch. You find these temptations are much easier to resist. You reach for your healthy lunch and go sit outside to soak up the sunshine.

7. Before long, you notice that your clothes fit differently and you feel better. You've lost a few pounds, have more energy, and feel happier. You see your doctor, who tells you to keep doing what you are doing and boosts your confidence that you are on the right track.

8. You have an "a-ha" moment: You see how it is all connected and you realize that you are now hooked on the Healthy Lifestyle Vortex! You wonder how and why it took you so long to switch from the old way to the new way. But then you trust that it's all part of your journey.

"A-Ha" Exercise

Healthy Lifestyle Vortex Exercise: Reflect on a recent experience where you fell off the healthy-eating wagon. Think about the three main triggers that contributed to your lapse. Of these triggers, choose the one that you could have controlled most easily. What would you have done differently? In what specific ways might a different choice in this one area have helped set a healthy vortex in motion, instead of an unhealthy one?

During the coming month, use the Healthy Lifestyle Vortex idea to help you build a case for going to the gym, having more vegetables at dinner, drinking less caffeine, and going to sleep earlier.

I'm Coaching Myself Thin!
CREATE A NEW WAY OF BEING

Tricia: "When I was in high school, I was always in the back of the line in PE. I was so shy and uncoordinated." She has now done several 5-Ks and admits that she's getting better at asking for help. Tricia has learned to look at her weight loss the same way she views building up her running stamina. "I take it a bit at a time, run a little farther each week, and keep moving forward," she says. "Even if I have to miss a run, I am not quitting. I am never to going to have it all together like I would like it to be, but that is okay. I need to make the best choices I can with what I have been given and not give up."

Jen: "I've been able to take some time to reflect on the journey I embarked on 5 years ago. I'm no longer that scared, unhappy, isolated person. I am stronger, I can do more than I ever thought possible, and I can do whatever I put my mind to. I've come to realize that my journey to weight loss is no longer about lowering cholesterol so I don't get put on medication. It isn't about what I look like or what others think about me. My journey to weight loss is about me—who I am, finding out what I am passionate about, and then having the energy and the health to do those things to the best of my ability. And it is a lifestyle that I plan to continue until the end."

PART 4

HEALTHY EATING GUIDELINES

CHAPTER 17

Nutrition Philosophy

Knowing what to eat can be very confusing. The commercials on TV tell you one thing and the "experts" tell you another. And the experts don't even agree on which foods are healthy: They all try to convince you that their plan will work the best, claiming to possess the missing piece of the weight-loss puzzle. But their plan may not work well for your individual needs and is not likely to be the missing piece from *your* particular puzzle. If you have the desire and are willing to make the effort, you can figure out what works best for you, much like a detective solves a mystery. The clues are provided by how you feel and how your body responds as you "clean up" your eating. While you won't get there overnight, you can only start where you're at and there's no time like right now to begin.

THE PROCESSED-FOOD INVASION

Aside from how advertisements influence and confuse you, the sheer number of food products available today is overwhelming. If you go into a regular supermarket, you'll see thousands of products on the shelves. But if you visit a small country store, you'll find only hundreds of products on the shelves. On closer inspection, you'll find the same staple foods that you would in the big supermarket: meats, fish, dairy products, grains, beans, fruits, and vegetables. What the smaller markets don't have are the dozen or so aisles of processed foods that take up the middle of the large markets. You know the products: They're in glossy packages and are designed more for taste and shelf life than good nutrition.

So why are these foods a problem? Let's pick on cheese puffs. In the right situation, you can argue that there is nothing at all wrong with them.

But if you really like cheese puffs—and even if they're not your favorite—you know how hard it is to stop eating them once a bag of them is open. If you sit down with that bag and watch a movie, it doesn't take long to inhale a shocking 800 calories' worth of these bright orange orbs. Science has shown through controlled studies that certain blends of salt, sugar, fat, and carbohydrates are almost addictive, a fact not lost on food companies who work diligently to create irresistible foods. (After all, their bottom lines depend on it.)

We believe that the idea that you "should" be able to keep your favorite snack foods around the house without overeating them is absurd. All it takes is one weak moment and the damage is done. And beating yourself up about your slip makes matters worse. If you want to make your nutrition program much easier for yourself, work on leaving your trigger foods on the supermarket shelves. This doesn't mean that you never get to eat another cheese puff if you really want one. The key is to develop a structure (see page 134) and be able to see where cheese puff calories can fit into it. If you are at a party and really want a few handfuls of cheese puffs, it may be the time to go for it! But to avoid the unnecessary temptation right out of the gate, keep them out of sight and out of mind.

Take a moment to think about your shopping habits and what you have in your pantry and refrigerator right now. If a supermarket *only* carried the foods you buy on a regular basis, and nothing else, what would it look like? Would there be aisles and aisles of chips, baked goods, and frozen dinners? Or would your supermarket look like the country store, selling mostly the whole foods that line the perimeter of the larger markets?

IT'S NOT SUPPOSED TO BE SO CONFUSING

Back in the day, our ancestors ate whole foods that they hunted and gathered from the fields, trees, forests, rivers, and oceans. In doing so, they nourished their bodies for optimal health.

A few thousand years ago, however, humans began hunting less and farming more, and as a result, new farm foods were introduced into our diet. Today, whole foods include lean meats (including wild game), seafood, dairy products (including milk, yogurt, and eggs), whole grains, nuts, seeds, beans, fruits, and vegetables.

As you may know, not all of these foods are digested well by everyone today. (If you need proof of this, look no further than the number of your friends who are intolerant to dairy or gluten.) Some experts make the case that we all should be eating only what the hunter-gatherers ate: meats, fruits, and vegetables. Other experts contend that many modern cultures with the longest life expectancies include grains and dairy products in their diets. The bottom line is that there is no one-size-fits-all diet. But there is one thing the experts do agree upon: Eating whole foods is the key to maintaining a healthy weight.

OVERFED AND UNDERNOURISHED

Millions of Americans are malnourished, despite getting plenty to eat. Marketers have sold us on the idea that it's good to eat fat-free, sugar-free, and low-calorie foods. Back when SnackWell's cookies were popular, researchers coined the phrase "the SnackWell Effect" to explain the phenomenon of overeating a low-calorie food and still not feeling physically satisfied. Beyond the psychological aspect of thinking you can "afford" to eat more because the food is low in calories, there is also a physical explanation: Empty calories from highly refined flours, fillers, and binders do not deliver the nutrients that satisfy your appetite. When you stick with whole foods, however, you will feel more satisfied on fewer calories. It's as simple as that.

MAKING THE TIME FOR HEALTHY FOOD

Let's face it: We're all sold on making our lives more convenient, and nothing is easier than getting food at a fast-food drive-through or ordering a pizza. A significant barrier to eating healthy for many is the time it takes to buy food, prepare it, cook it, and clean up afterwards. However, even if the mere thought of putting a healthy dinner on the table is exhausting, it's essential to focus on the payoffs—and the payoffs begin the first day that you make the time.

Would it increase your enjoyment of shopping and cooking if you *knew* that you were building better health as a result? Would redefining the kitchen cleanup tasks as "exercise" rather than "work" make it easier for you to burn a few more calories? If you don't yet have the cooking skills you would like to have or feel you need, would you be willing to start learning?

The answers to these questions may help you change your perspective. The truth is that you *are* building your health with every single meal, in the same way that a long journey is made up of single steps. Of the 1,000 meals you will eat in the coming year, imagine how much more energy you will have if you replace 80 percent of your less-healthy, on-the-go meals with balanced, home-prepared meals. And while cleaning your kitchen every night may be tiresome, the calories you burn doing so count every bit as much as those burned on a treadmill. And finally, you can become a dramatically better cook by getting in the kitchen with some good recipes and the guidance of a close friend or family member. We all learn through trial and error, so just get cooking and don't worry if some of your experiments are less delicious than others.

Before you worry that you need to become a chef and commit hours to shopping, preparing, cooking, and cleaning in order to eat healthfully, consider that what you really need is to become skilled at making healthy foods, whether that takes hours or just a few minutes. You can have quick *and* healthy, such as a turkey sandwich on whole wheat, along with hummus and some baby carrots. While the Quick Fix Mindset has conditioned you to choose microwaves, fast food, and convenience and to believe that food preparation is a hassle, consider that the opposite is possible for you: You may come to truly enjoy shopping for fresh foods and preparing them for yourself and your family.

GETTING ENOUGH

How do you know whether you're sticking to nature's design to maintain optimal health? To start with, here are three things you may be doing that mean you're *not*.

1. Eating artificial foods, including fat-free and sugar-free products, on a regular basis.
2. Taking supplements or other diet aids to suppress your appetite.
3. Skipping meals and snacks and ignoring your body's hunger signals.

You are working with nature's design when you choose a diet of whole foods, eat every 3 to 5 hours during the day, and give your body enough calories to support your resting metabolism and feel satisfied.

WEIGHT LOSS BY THE NUMBERS

Weight loss is quite simple, in theory: If you take in fewer calories than your body needs over a period of time, you'll lose weight. It doesn't matter if what you eat is nutritious or not; provided that you didn't exceed the number of calories you require, you could lose weight on a diet of potato chips and beer. And sadly, many place a greater value on weight loss than on their health and vitality. But this only speaks to how frustrated and desperate many are to lose weight so that they can feel better about how they look. If losing weight *and* building good health are your goals, then your plan needs to be health-promoting and packed with nutrient-dense whole foods right from the beginning. It has to accommodate your food preferences and be flexible enough to exclude those foods that disagree with you. You need to be able to modify your eating pattern based on your day-to-day life and to increase or decrease the amount of food you are eating based on feedback you're getting from your body. This plan needs to be your pride and joy, your way of life, and something you feel is your very own.

CHAPTER 18

Nutrition FAQ

What should I drink while trying to lose weight?

Since more than 60 percent of your body is made up of water, you need to drink 6 to 12 cups (48 to 96 ounces) of water each day for your body to function properly. After you meet your water needs, you can have other calorie-free or low-calorie beverages: sparkling water or club soda; black coffee or coffee with skim milk; herbal, black, or green tea; and artificially sweetened drinks (work to eliminate these beverages or at least limit to one daily until more is known about how artificial sweeteners affect appetite and overall metabolism). Caffeine is okay in moderation, but too much can cause irritability, poor sleep, and an energy crash late in the day. If you experience these effects, switch to decaf coffee or other caffeine-free beverages.

Tips for staying hydrated: Add freshly squeezed lemon or lime, fresh mint leaves, or a dash of 100 percent fruit juice to plain or sparkling water. Brew herbal teas and ice them at home, rather than buying bottled ice tea.

Fruit juice: While 100 percent fruit juice can be a healthy source of nutrients, it lacks fiber and is a concentrated source of calories and sugar. Limit yourself to 8 ounces per day or less.

Alcohol: Alcohol intake lowers inhibitions, which often leads to overeating and poor food choices. Plus, each drink (a 12-ounce beer, a shot of liquor, or a 5-ounce glass of wine) has 100 to 150 calories. These add up quickly if you consume several drinks, so keep alcohol to a minimum.

Why are there so many carbohydrates on the Coach Yourself Thin Eating Plan?

Because your brain and body require the blood sugar glucose, which comes from carbohydrates, you need quality carbohydrates in your diet. While refined carbohydrates—white flour, white rice, and refined sugars—can be problematic for blood sugar regulation, nature packages the essential nutrients you need for proper carbohydrate metabolism in the healthiest sources: whole grains, beans, vegetables, fruits, and dairy products. Many of our clients were convinced that they couldn't lose weight if they ate carbohydrates, but they discovered otherwise after building their eating plans around the carbohydrates listed as "Most Often" and greatly reducing or avoiding the "Sometimes" or "Infrequently" carbohydrates (see page 149). However, it is possible that your body will respond better to a diet that includes fewer carbohydrates, so you can modify your plan by replacing carbohydrate servings with calories from a lean protein or a healthy fat. If you have Type 2 diabetes, work with your doctor or certified diabetes educator to adjust your carbohydrate intake as needed.

What kind of bread should I buy?

When buying bread, look for the word "whole" on the ingredients list to identify products that contain whole wheat or other whole grains. Ingredients are listed in order of weight; thus a bread product has more whole grain flour than refined flour if whole wheat flour is listed before enriched flour. *Note:* Most commercial breads are made from white flour. Don't be fooled by the color of the packaging, a label indicating that the bread is multigrain or made from 100 percent wheat flour, or the addition of fiber to boost the fiber per slice. Look for breads that:

- List whole wheat flour before enriched wheat flour or, preferably, list whole wheat flour as the only flour.

- Contain at least 2 grams of fiber per 80 calories (usually about one slice). As mentioned above, bread makers add fiber to refined breads, but they do not add other important nutrients, such as vitamin E, magnesium, and selenium, all of which are found in the whole grain.

- Have a short list of ingredients that does not include preservatives. Ideally, your bread would be made of whole wheat flour, water, honey, yeast, and salt.

My digestive system is off—what can I do about it?

If you have recently increased your intake of fiber-rich fruits, vegetables, beans, and whole grains, your digestive processes will likely change. Though fiber typically loosens your stools, you may become constipated because of the abrupt change, and/or you may feel unusually full or bloated. Here's how to solve both problems.

Constipation: Drink at least six glasses of water each day and keep the amount of fiber in your plan consistent. If your fiber intake has been less than 20 grams per day on average, then you can achieve regularity by increasing your overall fiber intake from foods, such as a high-fiber cereal (containing more than 8 grams of fiber per serving) for breakfast, plus three or more servings of vegetables and two or three servings of fruit each day. If you become constipated *after* increasing your fiber significantly, then back off of concentrated fiber sources such as high-fiber cereals, fiber bars, or fiber supplements, but continue eating other fiber-rich foods (whole grains, vegetables, fruits, beans, nuts, and seeds). If constipation continues for another couple of days, try a psyllium-based fiber supplement to add bulk to your stool. (Follow the package directions.) You might also try 400 milligrams of magnesium citrate as a supplement; this mineral helps relax the smooth muscles, including the large intestine. Avoid taking magnesium within 2 hours of other medications, and do not take it if you have kidney disease. If constipation persists, consult with your doctor.

Gassiness and bloating: The short-term solution is to reduce or avoid high-fiber cereals, avoid fiber supplements, reduce the amount of raw vegetables in your diet, and reduce specific foods associated with gas production (apples, bananas, beans, peas, lentils, broccoli, Brussels sprouts, cabbage, cauliflower, corn, cucumbers, grapes, onions, raisins, and turnips). Do this until the gassiness and bloating subside. Slowly and systematically reintroduce these foods in the coming weeks, so your digestive system has a chance to adapt to your higher-fiber diet. In time, different types of bacteria will populate your digestive tract and your digestive function will improve significantly. You may still need to make certain amendments to improve digestibility, such as peeling your apples, cooking broccoli until it is soft, or avoiding raw cauliflower altogether.

I'm struggling with hunger. What should I do?

Ignoring hunger pangs won't work if you want to stick with your program for more than a few weeks. Start by making sure that you are eating enough calories to support your resting metabolism. (See the CYT calorie charts on pages 138 and 140 for guidance.) You should be eating three to six protein- and fiber-rich meals or snacks per day (your fiber intake should be at least 15 grams per 1,000 calories), but if you are still hungry, then you will need to increase your caloric intake by 200 to 300 calories per day. You can do this by adding 2 ounces of protein to your lunch or dinner, as well as an extra serving of vegetables and a serving of whole grains or beans.

One key strategy for managing hunger is to increase fiber intake because higher-fiber foods are more satisfying, calorie-for-calorie, than lower-fiber foods are. As a result, individuals with a higher fiber intake are more likely to have a lower body weight. The main food sources of fiber are high-fiber cereals, legumes (beans, lentils, and peas), fruits, vegetables, whole grains, and nuts and seeds.

Breakfast cereals: 0 to 13 grams of fiber per serving (read the label on the box to find the serving size)

Legumes (beans, lentils, and peas): 6 grams of fiber per ½ cup

Fruits, vegetables, and whole grains: 2 to 3 grams of fiber per serving (½ cup cooked veggies, 1 cup raw veggies, 1 slice whole wheat bread, 1 medium piece of fruit, ½ cup cut fruit, ¾ cup berries, 1 cup cubed melon, ½ cup oatmeal or brown rice)

Nuts and seeds: 2 grams of fiber per serving (1 small handful of nuts, 2 tablespoons peanut butter, 1 tablespoon ground flaxseed)

Should I buy all organic foods? I have a tight food budget and need to contain my expenses.

People choose organic foods to lower their intake of chemicals used in food production; to support farming practices that protect the farmers, the soil, and the water supply; and to improve conditions for farm animals. Now that organic farming is more commonly practiced, you can find organic foods at more reasonable prices in your local markets. However, if you need to prioritize your purchases to work within your budget, start with these affordable organic animal products: milk, yogurt, and eggs. You should also buy organically grown fruits and vegetables based on the "Dirty Dozen" (below). These twelve crops have been tested and found to contain roughly 90 percent of the pesticide residues found on all fruits and vegetables,[1] so it's well worth the extra money to buy organic.

Dirty Dozen

Apples	Nectarines (imported)	Blueberries (domestic)
Celery		
Strawberries	Grapes (imported)	Lettuce
Peaches	Sweet bell peppers	Kale/collard greens
Spinach	Potatoes	

Eco-Terms Defined

Organic: Plants and animals that have not been genetically modified (see definition below) and are grown or raised without the use of conventional pesticides or synthetic fertilizers; includes animal welfare standards and requires that feed is organically grown and does not contain synthetic additives (aside from trace minerals and vitamins) or animal byproducts.

Free-range, cage-free: Government regulations apply only to poultry. Free-range means that a hen has "access" to the outdoors, although this term is loosely regulated; the term "pastured" likely means greater outdoor access.

Hormone-free: Applies only to beef and milk because hormones are not permitted for use with pigs and chicken.

Genetically modified organism (GMO): A plant or animal whose genetic material has been altered using genetic engineering techniques.

How important are omega-3 fats? How can I get them if I don't eat fish?

There is a growing body of evidence that long-chain omega-3s offer some protection against coronary heart disease and may reduce overall inflammation in the body. The American Heart Association recommends eating fish at least two times per week, with an emphasis on fatty fish such as albacore tuna, anchovies, bluefish, herring, mackerel, salmon, and sardines. If you are not a fish eater, the other options for long-chain omega-3s are fish oil supplements or microalgae supplements. Discuss the supplement dosage with your doctor.

Your body can make some long-chain omega-3s from short-chain omega-3s, so include concentrated sources of these short-chain essential fats in your diet, as well: flaxseed or flaxseed oil, walnuts, non-GMO soy products (including tempeh and edamame), and non-GMO canola oil.

I'm not hungry in the morning and I don't want to eat when I'm not hungry. What should I do?

Not everyone has a strong appetite upon awakening. Keep in mind, though, that you will kick-start your metabolism by eating something healthy by midmorning at the latest and then eating a balanced meal or snack every 3 to 5 hours while you are awake. If that's not enough incentive and you're still not hungry, try having a light snack at breakfast, like a low-fat yogurt with a piece of fruit, and focus on consistency. Your body will soon adjust and you'll find your morning appetite, especially as you reduce or eliminate late-night eating.

Can I eat the same foods day after day and lose weight?

You can eat the same foods often and successfully lose weight, although the likelihood that you'll burn out and quit your program as a result increases significantly. Variety helps keep your food interesting and provides your body with essential nutrients, and some people need more variety than others do to be happy. Focus on adding more flavor to your food in a healthy way. According to Ayurveda, an ancient science of health and medicine, you derive all of the nutrients you need for optimal health when your meals contain all six tastes: sweet (like fruits and grains), sour (like yogurt), salty (like olives and feta cheese), bitter (like salad greens), pungent (like ginger and garlic), and astringent (like beans and pears). Consider simple ways to significantly enhance the flavor of your meals. For instance, try livening up your salads with one or more of these flavor enhancers: fresh basil, artichoke hearts, raisins, sautéed mushrooms, fresh parsley, toasted pecans, salsa, dried cranberries, caramelized onions, fresh jicama, or banana peppers.

You'll likely find that a small amount of a full-flavored food, such as freshly grated Parmesan, is much more satisfying than a larger portion of a reduced-fat food, such as part-skim mozzarella.

How do I eat out and still follow my program?

Follow these seven golden rules of eating out to become a master.

1. **Don't be *too* hungry when you go out or order takeout.** When you are starving, you are at a higher risk of making poor decisions, eating complimentary items like chips and bread, or ordering too much food and overeating.

2. **Have a plan.** Know exactly what you plan to order before sitting down. Map it out in your head, remind yourself of your program and your goals, and stick to your guns. Are you planning to have a drink or split a dessert? Follow this simple formula for ordering smart: Choose a moderate portion of lean protein, a big serving of vegetables, and a small serving of carbohydrates. Minimize the added fats by ordering dressing or sauce on the side. On special occasions, it's important to give yourself real permission to have something special without feeling guilty.

3. **Think big picture.** Remember that this is not your last supper and that another delicious meal is only a few hours away.

4. **Avoid all-you-can-eat specials, buffets, and situations that may tempt you to overeat.** With practice, you can learn to eat smart, but it takes discipline and now is the time to minimize unnecessary temptations.

5. **Control the immediate environment.** Ask that chips, bread, French fries, and other tempting restaurant foods be removed from the table, or at least move them away from you.

6. **Control your portions.** Split an entrée or visit restaurants that offer smaller portions. Given the size of portions in many American

restaurants, you may need to leave some food on your plate. One strategy is to order a clean plate and a take-home container at the start of the meal. Put only what you need on the plate and place the rest in the container to have for another meal. Take pride in your ability to turn delicious—yet excessive—food away.

7. **Enjoy every bite!** Eat slowly and appreciate your food by noticing its colors, textures, and aromas.

I'm short on time. How do I eat quickly and healthfully?

With practice, you can identify simple meals and snacks that are healthy, satisfying, and made from whole foods. Consider the following options, as well as those in the snack lists on page 154.

Sandwiches (Use 100 percent whole wheat bread or whole grain wraps with the following: peanut or almond butter and all-fruit jam, turkey, chicken breast slices, roast beef, tuna, egg salad, or a veggie burger. Use light mayonnaise or mustard.)

Salads from prewashed lettuce mixes, plus deli meat or rotisserie chicken, hard-boiled eggs, tuna, or cottage cheese

Whole grain cereal

Instant oatmeal, made from quick oats at home, with sunflower seeds, raisins, and cinnamon

Hard-boiled eggs

Baby carrots or celery sticks

Hummus

Whole foods–based energy bars

Low-fat granola bars

Apples, pears, bananas, or oranges

Nuts, measured into single-serving portions and stored in plastic baggies

Pineapple or peaches, canned in juice

Low-fat cottage cheese

Low-fat plain yogurt (Note: Flavored yogurt often contains 2 or 3 teaspoons of added sugar.)

Low-fat string cheese

Should I consider taking weight-loss supplements?

While supplements can produce weight loss, the effects are short-lived and can be detrimental to your health. Because an appetite suppressant isn't a lifestyle change, it's not a long-term plan for healthy weight loss. Spend your money on what is proven to work, will improve your health, and will help you be successful for years to come: quality whole foods.

What kinds of sweeteners are healthy? Are artificial sweeteners okay?

All sweeteners, including calorie-free sweeteners, can reduce the sensitivity of your taste buds to sweetness. This means that the more you use, the more you need in order to enjoy your food. By reducing your intake of sweeteners over a period of weeks, you can effectively heighten your sense of taste, allowing you to enjoy the subtle sweetness found in a variety of healthy foods.

For the sake of your health, use these no-calorie sweeteners little or not at all:

Artificial sweeteners: Reduce or avoid. It is not clear whether artificial sweeteners adversely affect metabolism and overall health. *Note:* If you are a diabetic, work with your doctor or diabetes educator to weigh the costs and benefits of artificial sweeteners.

Stevia: Made from leaves native to Brazil and Paraguay, stevia is an all-natural, calorie-free sweetener to choose instead of other calorie-free sweeteners. Use sparingly to minimize dulling your taste sensitivity or always needing your food to be sweetened.

Consume these sweeteners in small amounts, as needed:

Agave nectar (or agave syrup): Extracted from the blue agave plant, this liquid is sweeter than honey, although not as thick. It's sweeter than table sugar, as well, so you need less to achieve the same level of sweetness. One teaspoon has 20 calories.

Brown rice syrup: Made by cooking rice with enzymes to convert the starches into more simple sugars, brown rice syrup is not as sweet as table sugar and is absorbed into the bloodstream more slowly, making it easier for your body to maintain healthy blood sugar levels. One teaspoon has 13 calories.

Honey: This natural sweetener doesn't spoil and has antioxidant and antibacterial properties. Make the effort to find raw honey, which is absorbed more slowly into the bloodstream than pasteurized honey is. Local raw honey may also offer protection from allergies. One teaspoon has 21 calories.

Maple syrup: Derived from the sap of a variety of maple trees, maple syrup is categorized as grade A or grade B, based on the degree of processing. Grade B has slightly more nutrients and a stronger flavor. One teaspoon has 17 calories.

Turbinado sugar: Often called raw sugar, this cane sugar is not bleached or refined as much as white sugar. Plus, it contains molasses, which has manganese, copper, and iron in it. One teaspoon has 15 calories.

The scale isn't moving. What's going on?

The CYT program is designed to help you lose up to 1 percent of your body weight each week, although you may lose weight at a different rate. It is common to plateau for a few weeks after you lose 7 to 10 percent of your initial body weight. To overcome a plateau, eat enough to support your resting metabolism (see below), adjust your exercise program so that it remains challenging, strength-train three times each week, focus on your weekly goals, and remain patient and persistent. Your body may need an adjustment period of 2 to 3 weeks before resuming weight loss.

In the midst of a plateau, you may be inclined to cut calories further, but it is often the case that adding calories to better support your resting metabolism is the solution. The following explanation of how weight loss works will help you better understand where you can make changes to keep the scale moving.

Your body burns calories in three primary ways: through resting metabolism, daily activity, and exercise.

Resting metabolism rate (RMR): The number of calories burned by your body to stay alive and support the functioning of your vital organs is your RMR. Your RMR is responsible for roughly 70 percent of the total calories you burn. Most people's RMR is between 1,200 and 2,000 calories per day.

Daily activity: These are the calories you burn through moving your body each day as part of your normal activities, including walking and doing housework or yard work. Most people burn 300 to 600 daily activity calories per day, but this amount can be much higher for physical laborers.

Exercise. The calories burned by walking, swimming, biking, weight training, doing yoga, chopping wood, dancing, and so on. Most people burn 200 to 600 calories per workout.

If you don't eat enough calories to support your RMR, your body will burn additional muscle tissue for fuel, which drives down your metabolism. Your body can become surprisingly weight-loss resistant despite a low calorie intake, and this resistance can cause frustration. In these instances, adding 200 to 300 calories to your daily intake can help you overcome weight-loss resistance and get the scale moving again.

Here is a sample breakdown of daily calorie expenditure for an active person:

RMR: 1,500 calories

Daily activity: 600 calories

Exercise: 400 calories

Total calories expended in 24 hours: 2,500 calories

If this person ate 1,500 calories, she would have a 1,000-calorie daily deficit on exercise days and a 600-calorie deficit on rest days. Based on this estimate, she could anticipate a 1½- to 2-pound weekly weight loss (1 pound = 3,500 calories; a deficit of 1,000 calories per day x 6 days = 6,000 calories, plus a 600-calorie deficit x 1 day = 6,600 calories).

How do I estimate calories when I'm eating out or eating foods like a casserole?

It's not always easy to guesstimate the calories in your food, although with practice you can become proficient at estimating close enough. Start with common sense: Break the meal into carbohydrate portions (½ cup of pasta, rice, or potato or 1 slice of bread equals 80 to 100 calories), protein portions (each golf ball–size portion of meat or fish equals 40 to 80 calories, depending on the leanness), and fat portions (each tablespoon of oil has 120 calories; estimate 1 to 2 tablespoons for a restaurant-style entrée). Add up the portions and you'll have a reasonable estimate.

It would also help to familiarize yourself with what 1 cup of rice, lasagna, pasta, stew, etc., look like so that you are able to eyeball accurately. Do this when you're cooking at home, and you'll be able to estimate more accurately when you're out.

The following guide will help you estimate when a food is closer to 150 to 200 calories per cup than 300 to 400 calories per cup.

Soup, Stews, and Chili

Restaurant Soups

- Broth-based—200 calories per cup
- Cream-based—300 calories per cup

Home-Prepared or Canned Soups

- Tomato, vegetable, lentil, minestrone, chicken with rice, chicken vegetable—150 calories per cup
- New England–style clam chowder, cream of mushroom, bean with ham, cream of potato—200 calories per cup

Restaurant Stews

- Vegetarian—200 calories per cup
- Beef—300 calories per cup

Chili

- Vegetarian—200 calories per cup
- Beef and beans—300 calories per cup
- Beef, no beans—400 calories per cup

Lasagna and Casseroles

Lasagna

- Frozen—250 to 350 calories per cup
- Restaurant—400 calories per cup (standard restaurant portions is 2 cups)

Casseroles

- Vegetarian, no oil—200 calories per cup
- Vegetarian, light cheese or oil—250 calories per cup
- Meat-based, moderate fat—325 calories per cup
- Meat-based, higher fat—400 calories per cup

CHAPTER 19

Coach Yourself Thin Eating Plan Structure

We have developed the Coach Yourself Thin Eating Plan as a specific set of guidelines with an emphasis on:

Sustainability. Make your nutrition approach sustainable for the long-term by eating enough of the right types of foods to avoid hunger pangs, feelings of deprivation, and physical fatigue. Choose from all of the food groups as desired, establish consistent eating habits, and include treats to avoid burnout.

Nutrients. Choose quality whole foods that provide the essential nutrients needed for optimal health: lean meats (antibiotic-free and free-range, when possible), seafood, dairy products (including milk and yogurt), free-range eggs, whole grains, nuts and seeds, beans, fruits, and vegetables. Avoid or minimize consumption of fried foods, high-fat meats, refined flours, refined sugars (including high-fructose corn syrup), and processed foods that contain artificial sweeteners, hydrogenated oils, or chemical additives.

Your individual needs. Choose foods that work best for your digestion and taste preferences, and keep in mind any health issues you may have, such as diabetes, gluten sensitivity, or gastric reflux. Adjust your eating schedule and serving sizes to manage vacations, holidays, and sickness, and to overcome plateaus as necessary to help you stay on track.

GAUGING FULLNESS

Throughout the day and before and after each meal, take a moment to assess where you are on the Hunger and Fullness Scale.[1]

Hunger and Fullness Scale

1 = Very hungry; starving,

2 = Moderately hungry; ready to eat

3 = Mildly hungry

4 = Neutral, no sensations either way

5 = Mildly full. You feel satisfied

6 = Very full. Your stomach is beginning to feel a bit distended

7 = Much too full. Your stomach feels stuffed.

The goal is to *always* stay in the "desirable zone", a range from slightly hungrier than *mildly hungry* (2.5 on the scale) to a little more full than *mildly full* (5.5 on the scale). Avoid letting yourself get down to a 1 on the scale by keeping planned snacks on hand to eat if you fall below a 2.5. You'll begin to notice that when you are at 1 on the scale, you often end up at 6 or 7 because of poor food choices and over-eating.

BENEFITS OF COUNTING CALORIES

Tracking your calorie intake is the basis of the Coach Yourself Thin Eating Plan. It is the best way to ensure that you are not over- or under-eating your daily needs, and by following caloric guidelines, it's easier to be consistent from day to day. Think of calorie counting as a tool that can help you get on track, raise your awareness level, and help you identify the extra calories that make the difference between weight gain and weight loss. But let's be honest: Tracking calories isn't easy; there is no pedometer device for the tongue that does the work for you. It requires diligence and persistence. If you have a strong resistance to tallying your calories, try just writing your food intake down for 2 or 3 days and notice how this step influences your food choices. You may find that your resistance stems from feeling like you have to give up all of your favorite foods to be successful. If so, revisit the 80/20 Approach (see page 66) and think about how you can build some treats into your new program so you don't feel deprived.

Our goal for you is that you track calories only until you learn what you need to learn, you build confidence and trust in your ability to eat healthy most of the time, and you begin relying on your body's signals to regulate your intake. If you get stuck in a plateau or your weight begins to creep upwards, you can revisit calorie tracking, as needed, to help you get back in the driver's seat.

To get started with calorie counting, you'll need to educate yourself, using tools at home (such as a scale, measuring cups, and a measuring spoon), a dependable calorie counter, and the nutritional information on packaged food and restaurant Web sites (when available). There is a learning curve involved, but after a few weeks you will have memorized the calories in most of your favorite foods.

You've heard the saying, "Close only counts in horseshoes and hand grenades." Well, close also applies to calorie counting: You just need to consistently be within a couple hundred calories of your target to have weight-loss success. Keep in mind, however, that it is human nature to underestimate the actual calories consumed and, likewise, to overestimate the amount of exercise performed and calories expended.

The immediate goal of tracking calories is to help you find the *zone* where you are supporting your metabolic needs and feel satisfied, yet at the same time are in a calorie deficit so that you are steadily losing weight. When you sit down to your next meal or snack, you should be between a 2 and 3 on the Hunger Fullness Scale.

After you get started at a calorie level (which we will discuss on page 136) and are consistent for a few days, your body will become your guide. You will need to make modifications to your calorie intake based on your appetite and your energy levels, and how much and how hard you are exercising, as well as changes you see on the scale. If you have clear symptoms that you are not getting enough to eat, then you'll need to bump up your intake by at least one level. Do this for at least a week, and continue tuning in to the feedback you are getting.

Before bumping up your calories, however, first make sure that you are following the Eating Plan Design outlined below, particularly that you are distributing your calorie intake throughout the day and that you are reaching your fiber targets since both are necessary for balancing blood sugar and appetite and helping you feel more satisfied. If you are skipping meals or under-eating during the day, change your eating pattern so that you are consuming *half* of your daily calories during the first half of the day, and see how this makes it easier to be consistent.

Note: Psychologists do not recommend diets for those with severe emotional issues until their underlying emotions are resolved or the individual can effectively manage a weight-loss program. If you struggle with emotional eating, binge eating, anorexia, or another emotional disorder, we encourage you to find the necessary support you need, including guidance from an experienced psychotherapist. For a list of resources, see page 273.

EATING PLAN DESIGN

The following daily structures were designed to ensure that you:

1. Eat enough calories to support your resting metabolic needs.

2. Eat balanced meals comprised of healthy carbohydrates (vegetables, fruits, whole grains, and low-fat dairy), lean proteins, and healthy fats.

3. Eat a healthy meal or snack every 3 to 5 hours to balance out your appetite and blood sugar levels.

4. Choose *mostly* whole foods, with enough high-fiber choices so that you are getting at least 15 grams of fiber for every 1,000 calories you consume.

5. Stay adequately hydrated by consuming 6 to 12 cups of water daily.

6. Include a weekly treat budget as part of your program.

Your calorie recommendation is based on your gender, height, age, and current activity level. Select the appropriate gender chart (see pages 138 and 140) and identify your baseline diet level. There are 15 different calorie levels.

Next, review the activity criteria (see pages 139 and 141) and determine whether you need to make an upward adjustment to your diet level to accommodate your activity level. Finally, add or subtract a diet level (one diet level = 100 calories) depending on your current age (see below). It is easier physically and emotionally to add calories (rather than subtract them), so if you are not clear on the best level for you, start on the lower side and try it for a week. Assess your appetite and strength level, and adjust upward as needed.

CYT Calorie Levels for Women

To determine your overall diet level, find your starting level based on your current height—this is your baseline. Then adjust for your current body weight, and make any adjustments for activity and age as explained on the opposite page.

HEIGHT	LESS THAN 200 POUNDS (BASELINE LEVEL)	200–250 POUNDS	250–350 POUNDS	350 POUNDS OR MORE
4'10"	CYT 1,100	+100	+200	+300
4'11"	CYT 1,100	+100	+200	+300
5'0"	CYT 1,100	+100	+200	+300
5'1"	CYT 1,200	+100	+200	+300
5'2"	CYT 1,200	+100	+200	+300
5'3"	CYT 1,300	+100	+200	+300
5'4"	CYT 1,400	+100	+200	+300
5'5"	CYT 1,400	+100	+200	+300
5'6"	CYT 1,500	+100	+200	+300
5'7"	CYT 1,500	+100	+200	+300
5'8"	CYT 1,500	+100	+200	+300
5'9"	CYT 1,600	+100	+200	+300
5'10"	CYT 1,600	+100	+200	+300
5'11"	CYT 1,600	+100	+200	+300
6'0"	CYT 1,700	+100	+200	+300
6'1"	CYT 1,700	+100	+200	+300
6'2"	CYT 1,800	+100	+200	+300
6'3"	CYT 1800	+100	+200	+300
6'4"	CYT 1800	+100	+200	+300

Activity and Age Adjustment for Women

To help ensure that you are not overestimating your activity level, count only the minutes that you spend engaged in actual exercise, versus activities that are part of your normal daily life. (See page 131 for a definition of activities that are part of your normal daily life).

Weekly Exercise Minutes

0–150 minutes = No adjustment

150–240 minutes = Add 100 to your level

240–360 minutes = Add 200 to your level

360+ minutes = Add 300 to your level

Current Age

Under 25 years = Add 100 to your level

Over 50 years = Subtract 100 from your level

If you're on the borderline for either activity or age, start with the lower diet level and adjust upward later, if needed.

Diet Level = Baseline + Activity Adjustment +/- Age Adjustment

For example: A 43-year-old woman is 5'5" and weighs 145 pounds. She walks 30 minutes three times each week. Using the chart for women, her baseline level is CYT 1,500 with no activity adjustment and no age adjustment. A 24-year-old woman is 5'7" and weighs 231 pounds. She works out at the gym four times each week for 45 minutes on average. Using the chart for women, her baseline level is CYT 1,500 +100 to adjust for activity and +100 to adjust for age. Her final level is CYT 1,700.

CYT Calorie Levels for Men

To determine your overall diet level, find your starting level based on your current height–this is your baseline. Then adjust for your body weight, and make any adjustments for activity and age as explained below.

HEIGHT	LESS THAN 250 POUNDS (BASELINE LEVEL)	250–300 POUNDS	300–400 POUNDS	400+ POUNDS
5'0"	CYT 1,300	+100	+200	+300
5'1"	CYT 1,300	+100	+200	+300
5'2"	CYT 1,300	+100	+200	+300
5'3"	CYT 1,400	+100	+200	+300
5'4"	CYT 1,500	+100	+200	+300
5'5"	CYT 1,500	+100	+200	+300
5'6"	CYT 1,600	+100	+200	+300
5'7"	CYT 1,600	+100	+200	+300
5'8"	CYT 1,600	+100	+200	+300
5'9"	CYT 1,700	+100	+200	+300
5'10"	CYT 1,700	+100	+200	+300
5'11"	CYT 1,700	+100	+200	+300
6'0"	CYT 1,800	+100	+200	+300
6'1"	CYT 1,800	+100	+200	+300
6'2"	CYT 1,900	+100	+200	+300
6'3"	CYT 1,900	+100	+200	+300
6'4"	CYT 2,000	+100	+200	+300
6'5"	CYT 2,000	+100	+200	+300
6'6"	CYT 2,000	+100	+200	+300

Activity and Age Adjustment for Men

To help ensure that you are not overestimating your activity level, count only the minutes that you spend engaged in actual exercise, versus activities that are part of your normal daily life. (See page 131 for a definition of activities that are part of your normal daily life.)

Weekly Exercise Minutes

0–150 minutes = No adjustment

150–240 minutes = Add 100 calories to your level

240–360 minutes = Add 200 calories to your level

360+ minutes = Add 300 calories to your level

Current Age

Under 25 years = Add 100 calories to your level

Over 60 years = Subtract 100 calories from your level

If you're on the borderline for either activity or age, start with the lower diet level and adjust upward later, if needed.

Diet Level = Baseline + Activity Adjustment +/- Age Adjustment

For example: A 62-year-old man is 5'10" and weighs 255 pounds. He swims for 30 minutes three times each week. Using the chart for men, his baseline level is CYT 1,800, with no activity adjustment and an age adjustment of –100, for a final level of CYT 1,700. A 24-year-old male is 6'1" and weighs 210 pounds. He works out at the gym three times each week for an hour, on average. Using the chart for men, his baseline level is CYT 1,800, with an activity adjustment of +100 and an age adjustment of +100, for a final level of CYT 2,000.

Coach Yourself Thin Eating Plan Structure: 1,100–1,500 Calories

Locate your CYT Eating Plan Structure based on your diet level in the charts below. Each column contains the recommended servings of each food group for breakfast, lunch, a snack, and dinner. More information on servings of carbohydrates, protein, fat, fruits, vegetables, and calcium are described starting on page 149.

	CYT 1,100 CALORIES	CYT 1,200 CALORIES	
Breakfast	Carbs: 1 (80 calories)	Carbs: 1 (80 calories)	
	Protein: 1 oz (50 calories)	Protein: 1 oz (50 calories)	
	Fruit: 1 (60 calories)	Fruit: 1 (60 calories)	
	Fat: 1 (40 calories)	Fat: 1 (40 calories)	
	Total Calories: 230	Total Calories: 230	
Calcium / Dairy	–	1 (100 calories)	
Water	At least 16 oz	At least 16 oz	
Lunch	Carbs: 1 (80 calories)	Carbs: 1 (80 calories)	
	Protein: 2 oz (100 calories)	Protein: 2 oz (100 calories)	
	Vegetable: 2 (50 calories)	Vegetable: 2 (50 calories)	
	Fat: 1 (40 calories)	Fat: 1 (40 calories)	
	Total Calories: 270	Total Calories: 270	
Water	At least 16 oz	At least 16 oz	
Snack	200 calories	200 calories	
Dinner	Carbs: 2 (160 calories)	Carbs: 2 (160 calories)	
	Protein: 3 oz (150 calories)	Protein: 3 oz (150 calories)	
	Vegetable: 2 (50 calories)	Vegetable: 2 (50 calories)	
	Fat: 1 (40 calories)	Fat: 1 (40 calories)	
	Total Calories: 400	Total Calories: 400	
Actual Calories	**1,100**	**1,200**	

CYT 1,300 **CALORIES**	CYT 1,400 **CALORIES**	CYT 1,500 **CALORIES**
Carbs: 1 (80 calories)	Carbs: 1 (80 calories)	Carbs: 1 (80 calories)
Protein: 1 oz (50 calories)	Protein: 1 oz (50 calories)	Protein: 2 oz (100 calories)
Fruit: 1 (60 calories)	Fruit: 1 (60 calories)	Fruit: 1 (60 calories)
Fat: 1 (40 calories)	Fat: 1 (40 calories)	Fat: 1 (40 calories)
Total Calories: 230	Total Calories: 230	Total Calories: 280
1 (100 calories)	1 (100 calories)	1 (100 calories)
At least 16 oz	At least 16 oz	At least 16 oz
Carbs: 1 (80 calories)	Carbs: 2 (160 calories)	Carbs: 2 (160 calories)
Protein: 2 oz (100 calories)	Protein: 3 oz (150 calories)	Protein: 3 oz (150 calories)
Vegetable: 2 (50 calories)	Vegetable: 2 (50 calories)	Vegetable: 2 (50 calories)
Fat: 1 (40 calories)	Fat: 1 (40 calories)	Fat: 2 (80 calories)
Total Calories: 270	Total Calories: 400	Total Calories: 440
At least 16 oz	At least 16 oz	At least 16 oz
200 calories	200 calories	200 calories
Carbs: 2 (160 calories)	Carbs: 2 (160 calories)	Carbs: 2 (160 calories)
Protein: 4 oz (200 calories)	Protein: 4 oz (200 calories)	Protein: 4 oz (200 calories)
Vegetable: 2 (50 calories)	Vegetable: 2 (50 calories)	Vegetable: 2 (50 calories)
Fat: 2 (80 calories)	Fat: 2 (80 calories)	Fat: 2 (80 calories)
Total Calories: 490	Total Calories: 490	Total Calories: 490
1,290	**1,420**	**1,510**

Coach Yourself Thin Eating Plan Structure: 1,600–2,000 Calories

Locate your CYT Eating Plan Structure based on your diet level in the charts below. Each column contains the recommended servings of each food group for breakfast, lunch, a snack, and dinner. More information on servings of carbohydrates, protein, fat, fruits, vegetables, and calcium are described starting on page 149.

	CYT 1,600 CALORIES	CYT 1,700 CALORIES	
Breakfast	Carbs: 1 (80 calories)	Carbs: 1 (80 calories)	
	Protein: 2 oz (100 calories)	Protein: 2 oz (100 calories)	
	Fruit: 1 (60 calories)	Fruit: 1 (60 calories)	
	Fat: 1 (40 calories)	Fat: 1 (40 calories)	
	Total Calories: 280	Total Calories: 280	
Calcium / Dairy	1 (100 calories)	1 (100 calories)	
Water	At least 16 oz	At least 16 oz	
Lunch	Carbs: 2 (160 calories)	Carbs: 2 (160 calories)	
	Protein: 3 oz (150 calories)	Protein: 3 oz (150 calories)	
	Vegetable: 2 (50 calories)	Vegetable: 2 (50 calories)	
	Fat: 2 (80 calories)	Fat: 2 (80 calories)	
	Total Calories: 440	Total Calories: 440	
Water	At least 16 oz	At least 16 oz	
Snack	200 calories	300 calories	
Dinner	Carbs: 3 (240 calories)	Carbs: 3 (240 calories)	
	Protein: 4 oz (200 calories)	Protein: 4 oz (200 calories)	
	Vegetable: 2 (50 calories)	Vegetable: 2 (50 calories)	
	Fat: 2 (80 calories)	Fat: 2 (80 calories)	
	Total Calories: 570	Total Calories: 570	
Actual Calories	**1,590**	**1,690**	

CYT 1,800 CALORIES	CYT 1,900 CALORIES	CYT 2,000 CALORIES
Carbs: 2 (160 calories) Protein: 2 oz (100 calories) Fruit: 1 (60 calories) Fat: 1 (40 calories) Total Calories: 360	Carbs: 2 (160 calories) Protein: 2 oz (100 calories) Fruit: 1 (60 calories) Fat: 1 (40 calories) Total Calories: 360	Carbs: 2 (160 calories) Protein: 2 oz (100 calories) Fruit: 1 (60 calories) Fat: 1 (40 calories) Total Calories: 360
1 (100 calories)	1 (100 calories)	1 (100 calories)
At least 16 oz	At least 16 oz	At least 16 oz
Carbs: 2 (160 calories) Protein: 3 oz (150 calories) Vegetable: 2 (50 calories) Fat: 2 (80 calories) Total Calories: 440	Carbs: 2 (160 calories) Protein: 3 oz (150 calories) Vegetable: 2 (50 calories) Fruit: 1 (60 calories) Fat: 2 (80 calories) Total Calories: 500	Carbs: 3 (240 calories) Protein: 3 oz (150 calories) Vegetable: 2 (50 calories) Fruit: 1 (60 calories) Fat: 2 (80 calories) Total Calories: 580
At least 16 oz	At least 16 oz	At least 16 oz
300 calories	300 calories	300 calories
Carbs: 3 (240 calories) Protein: 4 oz (200 calories) Vegetable: 2 (50 calories) Fat: 2 (80 calories) Total Calories: 570	Carbs: 3 (240 calories) Protein: 4 oz (200 calories) Vegetable: 2 (50 calories) Fat: 3 (120 calories) Total Calories: 610	Carbs: 3 (240 calories) Protein: 5 oz (250 calories) Vegetable: 2 (50 calories) Fat: 3 (120 calories) Total Calories: 660
1,770	**1,870**	**2,000**

Coach Yourself Thin Eating Plan Structure: 2,100–2,500 Calories

Locate your CYT Eating Plan Structure based on your diet level in the charts below. Each column contains the recommended servings of each food group for breakfast, lunch, a snack, and dinner. More information on servings of carbohydrates, protein, fat, fruits, vegetables, and calcium are described starting on page 149.

	CYT 2,100 **CALORIES**	CYT 2,200 **CALORIES**	
Breakfast	Carbs: 2 (160 calories) Protein: 2 oz (100 calories) Fruit: 1 (60 calories) Fat: 1 (40 calories) Total Calories: 360	Carbs: 2 (160 calories) Protein: 2 oz (100 calories) Fruit: 2 (120 calories) Fat: 1 (40 calories) Total Calories: 420	
Calcium / Dairy	1 (100 calories)	1 (100 calories)	
Water	At least 16 oz	At least 16 oz	
Lunch	Carbs: 3 (240 calories) Protein: 3 oz (150 calories) Vegetable: 2 (50 calories) Fruit: 1 (60 calories) Fat: 2 (80 calories) Total Calories: 580	Carbs: 3 (240 calories) Protein: 4 oz (200 calories) Vegetable: 2 (50 calories) Fruit: 1 (60 calories) Fat: 2 (80 calories) Total Calories: 630	
Water	At least 16 oz	At least 16 oz	
Snack	300 calories	300 calories	
Dinner	Carbs: 4 (320 calories) Protein: 5 oz (250 calories) Vegetable: 2 (50 calories) Fat: 3 (120 calories) Total Calories: 740	Carbs: 4 (320 calories) Protein: 5 oz (250 calories) Vegetable: 2 (50 calories) Fat: 3 (120 calories) Total Calories: 740	
Actual Calories	**2,080**	**2,190**	

CYT 2,300 CALORIES	CYT 2,400 CALORIES	CYT 2,500 CALORIES
Carbs: 2 (160 calories) Protein: 2 oz (100 calories) Fruit: 2 (120 calories) Fat: 1 (40 calories) Total Calories: 420	Carbs: 2 (160 calories) Protein: 2 oz (100 calories) Fruit: 2 (120 calories) Fat: 1 (40 calories) Total Calories: 420	Carbs: 2 (160 calories) Protein: 2 oz (100 calories) Fruit: 2 (120 calories) Fat: 2 (80 calories) Total Calories: 460
1 (100 calories)	1 (100 calories)	1 (100 calories)
At least 16 oz	At least 16 oz	At least 16 oz
Carbs: 3 (240 calories) Protein: 4 oz (200 calories) Vegetable: 2 (50 calories) Fruit: 1 (60 calories) Fat: 2 (80 calories) Total Calories: 630	Carbs: 3 (240 calories) Protein: 4 oz (200 calories) Vegetable: 2 (50 calories) Fruit: 1 (60 calories) Fat: 3 (120 calories) Total Calories: 670	Carbs: 4 (320 calories) Protein: 4 oz (200 calories) Vegetable: 2 (50 calories) Fruit: 1 (60 calories) Fat: 2 (80 calories) Total Calories: 710
At least 16 oz	At least 16 oz	At least 16 oz
300 calories	300 calories	300 calories
Carbs: 4 (320 calories) Protein: 7 oz (350 calories) Vegetable: 2 (50 calories) Fat: 3 (120 calories) Total Calories: 840	Carbs: 5 (400 calories) Protein: 6 oz (300 calories) Vegetable: 2 (50 calories) Fat: 4 (160 calories) Total Calories: 910	Carbs: 5 (400 calories) Protein: 6 oz (300 calories) Vegetable: 2 (50 calories) Fat: 4 (160 calories) Total Calories: 910
2,290	**2,400**	**2,480**

On occasions when you are unable to closely follow your Coach Yourself Thin Eating Plan Structure, refer to the chart below and find your diet level so that you can aim to meet the calorie targets for each meal and snack. Use any available nutritional information plus your own knowledge to estimate your intake. This approach is ideal when you are out of your normal routine, such as on vacation or traveling for business. To help you stay on track throughout the day, copy the chart below to have your calorie targets on hand.

CALORIE	BREAKFAST	LUNCH	SNACK	DINNER	TOTAL
CYT 1,100	230	270	200	400	1,100
CYT 1,200	300	300	200	400	1,200
CYT 1,300	300	300	200	500	1,300
CYT 1,400	300	400	200	500	1,400
CYT 1,500	350	450	200	500	1,500
CYT 1,600	350	450	200	600	1,600
CYT 1,700	350	450	300	600	1,700
CYT 1,800	450	450	300	600	1,800
CYT 1,900	450	500	300	650	1,900
CYT 2,000	450	600	300	650	2,000
CYT 2,100	450	600	300	750	2,100
CYT 2,200	500	650	300	750	2,200
CYT 2,300	500	650	300	850	2,300
CYT 2,400	500	650	300	950	2,400
CYT 2,500	500	750	300	950	2,500

To help you stay balanced, use the following meal and snack guidelines.

Breakfast: Include a small serving of a high-fiber carbohydrate + lean protein + small amount of healthy fat + calcium/dairy + fruit

Lunch: Include a small serving of a high-fiber carbohydrate + lean protein + small amount of healthy fat + vegetables

Snack: Healthy whole foods snack based on nuts, seeds, low-fat dairy, fruits, vegetables, or other whole foods

Dinner: Include a small serving of a high-fiber carbohydrate + lean protein + small amount of healthy fat + vegetables

Carbohydrate Guide

When you are reading the Nutrition Facts label on a packaged food, keep in mind that one carbohydrate serving equals 15 grams of carbohydrates, or approximately 80 calories. The following chart shows you the types of carbohydrates to eat Most Often, Sometimes, or Infrequently.

MOST OFTEN	Whole wheat bread, brown rice, high-fiber cereals, oatmeal, quinoa, beans (including peas and edamame), hummus, sweet potatoes, corn, millet, winter squash, whole wheat pasta, 100 percent whole grain crackers, wild rice, air-popped popcorn, and other whole grains. *Note:* Other healthy carbohydrates to eat regularly include vegetables, fruits, and low-fat dairy products (discussed later in this chapter).
SOMETIMES	All refined white flour breads, including but not limited to pita bread, sandwich bread, French bread, English muffins, tortillas, dinner rolls, and bagels; white flour pancakes and waffles; low-fiber cereals; white rice; refined pasta; baked potatoes; pizza; and pretzels.
INFREQUENTLY	Sugary cereals, biscuits, mashed potatoes, cakes, doughnuts, cookies, pastries, French fries, soft drinks, juice drinks, and candy.

"Most Often" Carbohydrates (serving size = approximately 80 calories)

- 1 ounce whole wheat and other 100 percent whole grain bread (3 or more grams of fiber per 80-calorie serving)
- ½ cup cooked or 1 ounce dry whole wheat pasta (at least 50 percent whole grain)
- 1 ounce whole grain crackers (at least 3 grams of fiber per serving)

- 3 ounces baked sweet potato (¼ large potato)
- Heaping ⅓-cup portion cooked brown rice, quinoa, or millet
- Higher-fiber breakfast cereals (at least 3 grams of fiber; see labels for serving sizes)
- ½ cup cooked oatmeal
- ½ cup black beans, kidney beans, garbanzo beans, peas, or other legumes
- 3 cups air-popped popcorn
- 1 cup cooked acorn squash, butternut squash, Hubbard squash, pumpkin, or spaghetti squash
- 3 tablespoons low-fat hummus
- ½ cup cooked amaranth
- ½ cup cooked wild rice

"Sometimes" Carbohydrates (serving size = approximately 80 calories)

- 1 ounce bread (typically one slice; see labels for serving sizes)
- ½ cup cooked or 1 ounce dry pasta
- 6 saltine crackers
- 3 ounces baked potato (¼ large potato)
- ⅓ cup white rice
- ¾ cup most breakfast cereals (see label to determine 80-calorie amount)
- 1 ounce bagel (½ small bagel or ⅓ deli bagel)
- ½ English muffin

Protein Guide

When you are reading the Nutrition Facts label on a packaged food, keep in mind that 1 ounce of protein is equal to 7 grams of protein. The target for protein is 50 calories or fewer per ounce. If your protein choices have more than 50 calories per ounce, adjust your portions as needed to stay within your calorie target.

One ounce of protein (prepared with no added fats) equals 1 ounce by weight and is approximately the size of a golf ball, unless otherwise specified. For reference, a 3-ounce serving is about the size of a deck of cards. The following chart shows you the types of protein to eat Most Often, Sometimes, or Infrequently.

MOST OFTEN	Protein sources that contain 50 calories or fewer per 6 to 7 grams of protein (50 calories per ounce or less), including chicken breast; skinless turkey breast; low-fat or nonfat cottage cheese (¼ cup); 3 egg whites; all wild game; fish (not fried), including salmon, cod, flounder, sardines, and all white fish. Plant proteins: 1 oz tempeh (50 calories), ½ cup beans (100 calories), ½ cup peas (60 calories), and ¼ cup edamame (60 calories).
SOMETIMES	Protein sources that contain less than 75 calories per ounce, including fish (tuna and other mercury-containing fish*), shellfish, and catfish; chicken thigh or leg (skinless); ground chicken or turkey breast; egg(choose cage-free); flank steak; lean roast beef; top and round cuts of beef; trimmed filet mignon; pork tenderloin; boiled ham (low-sodium); lean and extra-lean ground beef (90% lean or leaner); lean Canadian bacon, and other lean cuts of red meat. *Note:* Choose "Select" grade and grass-fed meats when possible. Low-fat cheese, part-skim string cheese, full-fat cheese (90–120 calories per ounce), in small amounts. Plant proteins: 2 oz extra-firm tofu (50 calories), ½ veggie burger patty (see label), 1 oz veggie sausage (50 calories), or 1 veggie hot dog (see label).
INFREQUENTLY	Protein sources that contain 75 or more calories per ounce, including fried chicken, chicken and turkey with skin, ground chicken or turkey (including skin and dark meat), fried fish, prime rib, ground beef (90% lean or less), hot dogs, sausage, bacon, pepperoni, salami, bratwurst, organ meats, and other higher-fat red meats or processed meats.

Note: Be aware of your intake of fish containing higher levels of mercury, such as tuna, grouper, orange roughy, and king mackerel. For more information, visit www.gotmercury.org.

Fruit Guide

A typical serving of fruit has 60 calories and 15 grams of carbohydrates. Here is a list of single-serving options.

4-ounce apple (tennis ball–size)

½ cup applesauce

4 dried apple rings

4 whole apricots

8 dried apricot halves

½ large banana

¾ cup blackberries

¾ cup blueberries

1 cup cantaloupe cubes

12 sweet cherries

3 dates

1½ large fresh figs

1½ dried figs

½ cup fruit cocktail

½ large grapefruit

17 small grapes

1 cup honeydew cubes

1 kiwifruit

½ cup mango

1 small nectarine

1 medium orange

1 cup papaya cubes

1 medium peach

½ cup canned peaches

1 medium pear

¾ cup fresh pineapple

½ cup canned pineapple

2 small plums

3 prunes

2 tablespoons raisins

1 cup raspberries

¾ cup sliced strawberries

2 small tangerines

1¼ cups watermelon cubes

Note: Fruit juice contains a lot of sugar and calories and dried fruit lacks water content, making it calorie-dense. Minimize your intake of fruit juice and dried fruit while you're trying to lose weight.

Vegetable Guide

A typical serving of vegetables has 25 calories and 5 grams of carbohydrates. A standard serving is ½ cup of cooked vegetables, 1 cup of raw vegetables, or 2 cups of salad greens. Here is a list of vegetables to select from while you follow the Coach Yourself Thin Eating Plan.

Artichoke hearts, 2 pieces

Asparagus

Beans (green, wax, or Italian)

Bean sprouts

Beets

Broccoli

Brussels sprouts

Cabbage

Carrots

Cauliflower

Celery

Cucumbers

Eggplant

Green onions

Greens (collard, kale, mustard, turnip, or Swiss chard)

Jicama, ½ cup raw

Kohlrabi

Leeks

Lettuce (iceberg, romaine, green leaf, or red leaf)

Mixed salad greens, including arugula, radicchio, escarole, endive, and spinach

Mushrooms

Okra

Onions

Pea pods

Peppers

Radishes

Sauerkraut (limit to ½-cup serving because of high sodium content)

Spinach

Summer squash (yellow)

Tomato, 2 large slices

Tomato sauce, ½ cup

Turnips

Water chestnuts, ¼ cup slices

Zucchini

Fats Guide

A typical serving of fat is 5 grams and contains 40 calories. The following chart shows you the types of fat to eat Most Often, Sometimes, or Infrequently.

MOST OFTEN	Avocado, extra-virgin olive oil, canola oil (non-GMO), olives, nuts (unsalted), seeds (unsalted), nut and seed butters, nut- or tahini-based creamy salad dressing, olive oil–based dressing, sesame oil, and organic ghee.
SOMETIMES	Vegetable oil, low-fat mayonnaise, organic butter, virgin coconut oil, coconut milk, coconut (fresh or dried), grapeseed oil, light olive oil, and low-fat salad dressing (commercial brands).
INFREQUENTLY	Regular mayonnaise, margarine (trans-fat free), and oil-based creamy salad dressing.

One standard serving of fat is:

1 teaspoon any oil

1 teaspoon regular mayonnaise

1 tablespoon low-fat mayonnaise

1 teaspoon butter or margarine

2 teaspoons creamy salad dressing

1 tablespoon low-fat salad dressing

⅙ avocado

5 medium olives

6 whole almonds

2 whole Brazil nuts

5 whole cashews

3 macadamia nuts

1 tablespoon mixed nuts, unsalted

7 whole peanuts

4 pecans halves

10 shelled pistachios

3 walnut halves

1 tablespoon flaxseed, ground

2 teaspoons pumpkin seeds, unsalted

1 tablespoon sunflower seeds, unsalted

2 teaspoons sesame seeds, toasted

1 teaspoon nut or seed butter (peanut, almond, cashew, sunflower, or tahini)

Note: Nuts and seeds provide essential nutrients and satisfaction, and you are encouraged to eat them as part of your meals and everyday snacks. Because they are calorie-dense and easy to overconsume, make it a rule to always eat them with a lower-calorie food such as fruit, vegetables, low-fat yogurt, or whole-grain cereal, or mix a premeasured quantity into a salad or stir-fry.

Calcium/Dairy Guide

A typical serving of dairy or a calcium-fortified nondairy substitute has 110 calories or fewer and provides 200 milligrams or more of calcium per serving. Choose from:

1 cup nonfat or 1 percent milk, preferably organic

1 cup unsweetened almond milk, enriched

1 cup nonfat soy milk, enriched

1 cup plain rice milk, enriched

6 ounces (1 container) nonfat plain yogurt

6 to 8 fluid ounces 100 percent orange juice with added calcium

Condiments Guide

Low-calorie condiments can add flavor and variety to your meals. Keep track of the calories in your condiments and use them in place of other calories, such as a fat serving (40 calories). Choose from the following list of salad dressings and other condiments while eating to lose weight.

SALAD DRESSING	CALORIES
Fat-free Italian (2 Tbsp)	10
Reduced-fat balsamic or red wine vinaigrette (2 Tbsp)	40
Light honey Dijon (2 Tbsp)	50
Light Italian (2 Tbsp)	50
OTHER CONDIMENTS	**CALORIES**
Spice blends, sodium-free (1 Tbsp)	0
Hot sauce (1 Tbsp)	0
Dill relish (1 Tbsp)	0
Mustard: yellow, Dijon, stone ground, and spicy brown (1 Tbsp)	0
Vinegars: balsamic, rice, and wine (1 Tbsp)	0
Lemon or lime juice (1 Tbsp)	0
Bragg Liquid Aminos or reduced-sodium tamari sauce (1 tsp)	3–5
Picante sauce (1 Tbsp)	5
Wasabi paste (1 tsp)	15
Ketchup (1 Tbsp)	15–20
Salsa (1 Tbsp)	10–15
BBQ sauce (see label)	10–20
Jam/jelly (see label)	15–60
Light sour cream (1 Tbsp)	20
Parmesan cheese (1 Tbsp)	25
Marinara sauce (¼ cup)	25
Light cream cheese (1 Tbsp)	30
Pickles, sweet (6 slices)	30
Tofu-based mayonnaise (1 Tbsp)	35
Low-fat mayonnaise (1 Tbsp)	40

Snacks

A 200- to 300-calorie midafternoon snack will help balance your blood sugar levels and appetite, making it easier to eat moderately during the evening. Here are examples of healthy snacks to put together.

200-Calorie Snacks—Nut and Fruit Combos

Choose any nut portion on the left column to eat with any fruit portion on the right column.

NUT PORTION = 140 CALORIES	+	FRUIT PORTION = 60 CALORIES	TOTAL CALORIES
20 almonds		4 oz apple	**200**
15 medium cashews		½ cup applesauce	**200**
6 medium Brazil nuts		½ regular banana	**200**
8 macadamia nuts		¾ cup blueberries	**200**
35 pistachios		1 kiwifruit	**200**
10 walnut halves		½ cup cubed mango	**200**
14 pecan halves		1 small nectarine	**200**
1 heaping Tbsp peanut butter		1 medium orange	**200**
1 heaping Tbsp almond butter		1 medium peach	**200**
24 dry-roasted peanuts		½ cup canned peaches	**200**
		½ large pear	**200**
		¾ cup fresh pineapple chunks	**200**
		½ cup canned pineapple chunks	**200**
		2 small plums	**200**
		1 cup raspberries	**200**
		1 cup sliced strawberries	**200**
		1 large tangerine	**200**

Other 200-Calorie Snacks

						TOTAL CALORIES
1 slice whole grain toast (3+ grams fiber per slice)	100	3 Tbsp low-fat hummus	75	2 slices tomato	20	**195**
15 large baby carrots	75	1 cup broccoli florets	30	5 oz low-fat plain yogurt mixed with herbs	90	**195**
3 oz canned light tuna in water	100	½ slice whole grain toast (3+ grams fiber per slice)	50	1 Tbsp light mayonnaise	50	**200**
1 hard-boiled egg	70	½ whole wheat English muffin	70	1 Tbsp light mayonnaise	50	**190**
3 slices turkey breast lunch meat	65	6 whole grain crackers	75	1 Tbsp light mayonnaise	50	**190**
½ cup nonfat fruit yogurt	100	7 almonds	50	½ cup raspberries	30	**180**
1 hard-boiled egg	70	5 low-fat whole wheat crackers (3+ grams fiber per serving)	90	2 tsp light mayonnaise	30	**190**
Veggie burger (soy or bean-based)	130	1 slice low-fat American cheese	40	Pickles, ketchup, and mustard	25	**195**
1 cup oatmeal	160	1 Tbsp raisins	30	1 tsp brown sugar	20	**210**
1 slice whole grain toast (3+ grams fiber per slice)	100	¼ avocado	80	1 slice tomato	10	**190**
Greek Salad: 2 cups sliced tomato and cucumber	35	Dressing: balsamic vinegar, 2 tsp olive oil, 1 spray Bragg Liquid Aminos	90	4 whole grain crackers	50	**175**
4 cups fresh spinach greens	30	Dressing: balsamic vinegar, 2 tsp olive oil, 1 spray Bragg Liquid Aminos	90	6 whole grain crackers	75	**195**
½ cup shredded carrots, ½ cup shredded beets, and 1 Tbsp raisins	85	Dressing: 1 Tbsp balsamic vinaigrette (bottled)	45	Pecans, toasted, 7 halves	70	**200**

(continued)

						TOTAL CALORIES
5 stalks of celery, 5" long	10	1 cup low-fat or nonfat cottage cheese	160	Pineapple, ¼ cup crushed	35	**205**
100% fruit popsicle	50	20 almonds	140			**190**
4 whole grain crackers	50	1 Tbsp + 1 tsp peanut butter	140			**190**
3 cups air-popped popcorn	90	1 Tbsp butter	100			**190**
3 Tbsp low-fat hummus	75	7 low-fat whole wheat crackers (3+ grams fiber per serving)	125			**200**
6 low-fat whole wheat crackers (3+ grams fiber per serving)	110	1 Tbsp reduced-fat peanut butter	95			**205**
¾ cup pineapple chunks in juice	90	½ cup low-fat or nonfat cottage cheese	80			**170**
Nonfat or low-fat granola bar (3+ grams fiber and 3 or fewer grams fat)	120	1 small apple	75			**195**
¾ cup bran cereal	120	¾ cup skim milk or fortified low-fat soy milk	65			**185**
¼ cup soy nuts	120	1 small apple	75			**195**
2 cups sliced strawberries	120	2 Tbsp chocolate syrup	70			**190**
1 cup canned or instant lentil or split pea soup	150	4 whole grain crackers	50			**200**
1 cup chicken rice, tomato, or mushroom soup	150	4 whole grain crackers	50			**200**
¾ cup green soybeans	150	¼ cup light soy sauce	40			**190**
1 regular frozen banana	120	12 almonds	80			**200**

							TOTAL CALORIES
1 mini-box raisins	42	22 almonds	155				**197**
2 whole rye crackers	80	¾ cup low-fat or nonfat cottage cheese	120				**200**
4 slices turkey breast lunch meat	90	3 Tbsp jellied cranberry sauce	80				**170**
12 small shrimp	120	¼ cup cocktail sauce	60				**180**
15 baby carrots	75	4 Tbsp low-fat hummus	100				**175**
2 medium cucumbers, sliced	60	8 oz low-fat plain yogurt mixed with herbs	140				**200**
1 large tomato, sliced, with 1 oz fresh part-skim mozzarella	105	Dressing: balsamic vinegar, 2 tsp olive oil, 1 spray Bragg Liquid Aminos	90				**195**
4 cups salad greens and 1 cup cucumber	50	2 Tbsp tahini dressing	140				**190**
2 whole grain rice cakes	70	⅓ avocado	105				**175**
1 cup nonfat yogurt	140	1 cup sliced strawberries	60				**200**
1 medium apple	95	¼ cup brown rice, ½ tsp cinnamon, and 1 Tbsp raisins	90				**185**
3 Nori Wraps: Nori seaweed sheet rolled with 2 tsp hummus, slivered cucumber, shredded carrot, sprouts	180						**180**
1 medium apple	95	¼ cup brown rice, ½ tsp cinnamon, 1 Tbsp raisins, 3 walnuts halves	120				**215**

300-Calorie Snacks—Nut and Fruit Combos

Choose any nut portion on the left column to eat with any fruit portion on the right.

NUT PORTION = 180 CALORIES	+	FRUIT PORTION = 120 CALORIES	TOTAL CALORIES
26 almonds		1 large apple	300
20 medium cashews		1 cup applesauce	300
8 medium Brazil nuts		8 dried apple rings	300
10 macadamia nuts		1 medium banana	300
45 pistachios		1¾ cups blackberries	300
13 walnut halves		1½ cups blueberries	300
18 pecan halves		1 cup fruit cocktail	300
1 Tbsp + 2 tsp peanut butter		1 large grapefruit	300
1 Tbsp + 2 tsp almond butter		35 small grapes	300
30 peanuts		2 kiwifruits	300
		1 cup cubed mango	300
		2 small nectarines	300
		1 large orange	300
		2 medium peaches	300
		1 cup canned peaches	300
		1 large pear	300
		1½ cups fresh pineapple chunks	300
		1 cup canned pineapple chunks	300
		4 small plums	300
		2 cups raspberries	300
		2 cups sliced strawberries	300
		2 large tangerines	300

Other 300-Calorie Snacks

							TOTAL CALORIES
2 cups sliced strawberries	120	1 cup blueberries	85	2 Tbsp chocolate syrup	70		275
1 cup nonfat yogurt	140	13 almonds	90	1 cup raspberries	60		290
1 cup green soybeans (edamame)	200	4 whole grain saltine crackers	50	⅓ cup light soy sauce	50		300
3 oz canned light tuna in water	100	1½ slices whole grain toast (3+ grams fiber per slice)	150	1 Tbsp light mayonnaise	50		300
2 hard-boiled eggs	140	1 slice whole grain toast (3+ grams fiber per slice)	100	1 Tbsp light mayonnaise	50		290
1 cup bran cereal	190	½ medium banana	60	½ cup skim milk or fortified low-fat soy milk	45		295
1¼ cups oatmeal	200	2 Tbsp raisins	60	2 tsp brown sugar	40		300
2 slices whole grain toast (3+ grams fiber per slice)	200	⅓ avocado	105	1 slice tomato	10		315
½ cup soy nuts	240	½ medium banana	60				300
1½ cups pineapple chunks in juice	180	¾ cup nonfat cottage cheese	120				300
4 fig bars	220	1 small apple	75				295
6 cups air-popped popcorn	180	1 Tbsp flax, canola, or olive oil	120				300
6 cups air-popped popcorn	180	1 Tbsp butter	100				280
1 cup canned or instant lentil or split pea soup	150	12 whole grain saltine crackers	150				300

(continued)

						TOTAL CALORIES
4 Tbsp low-fat hummus	120	10 low-fat whole wheat crackers (3+ grams fiber per serving)	180			**300**
Low-fat granola bar (3+ grams fiber and 3 or fewer grams fat)	180	1 large apple	120			**300**
8 whole grain saltine crackers	100	2 Tbsp peanut butter	200			**300**
2 fruit popsicles, 100% fruit	100	27 almonds	190			**290**

WEEKLY TREAT BUDGET

You are encouraged to have a significant treat each week, if you wish. If your regular daily snack is 200 calories, then have a 400-calorie treat of your choice once each week; if your daily snack is 300 calories, have a 600-calorie treat, or divide it up throughout the week as desired. Choose anything—the only rules are that it is a guilt-free treat you enjoy and that you give yourself this treat with full permission *as part of* your weight-loss program.

SHOPPING LIST

The following shopping list will help you stock your kitchen with a variety of healthy foods. Spend a few minutes taking inventory of the foods that you like. Then create your own shopping list and keep it in your wallet to use the next time you go shopping for food.

Dairy and Nondairy Substitutes (Protein and Calcium)

Eggs (cage-free or free-range), egg whites (packaged), nonfat milk or 1 percent milk (preferably organic), unsweetened almond milk, nonfat enriched soy milk, enriched plain rice milk, low-fat plain yogurt, low-fat or nonfat cottage cheese, low-fat sour cream, low-fat cream cheese, low-fat cheese (mozzarella, Cheddar, pepper jack, etc.), feta cheese, goat cheese, Parmesan, and Romano.

Meat, Chicken, and Fish (Lean Protein)

Red meat: Lean Canadian bacon, lean or extra-lean ground beef (at least 96 percent lean), sliced boiled ham (low-sodium), sliced roast beef (low-sodium), lean pork tenderloin, venison, wild game of any type.

Chicken and turkey: Skinless chicken and turkey breasts, lean or extra-lean ground chicken breast, lean or extra-lean ground turkey breast.

Fish and shellfish: Tuna (canned in water, solid white or chunk light), cod, halibut, flounder, lobster, canned wild salmon, salmon, tilapia, sardines, sea bass, swordfish, shrimp.

Vegetables and Fruits

Vegetables: Asparagus, avocado, bell peppers (red, yellow, orange, green), chile peppers, broccoli, Brussels sprouts, carrots, cauliflower, celery, cherry tomatoes, collard greens, corn, cucumbers, eggplant, garlic, green beans, jicama, kale, lettuce (all kinds), mushrooms, onions, radishes, spaghetti squash, spinach (fresh or frozen), summer squash (yellow), winter squash (butternut, acorn, Hubbard), tomatoes, zucchini.

Fruits: Apples (all kinds), bananas, blackberries, blueberries, cherries, grapefruit, kiwifruit, lemons, mangoes, melons, nectarines, oranges (all kinds), papayas, peaches, pears, pineapple, plums, raspberries, strawberries.

Beans and Legumes

Dry or low-sodium canned: Aduki, black, pinto, garbanzo, kidney, great northern, lima, and mung beans; black-eyed peas, split peas, lentils.

Cereals, Grains, and Breads

Breakfast cereals: Bran cereals with 8 or more grams of fiber per serving, old-fashioned oats, shredded wheat; gluten-free hot cereals including quinoa flakes, brown rice flakes, and cream of buckwheat.

Grains: Brown rice, brown rice pasta, bulgur, millet, popcorn (whole kernels, not microwave popcorn with added flavorings), whole wheat couscous, whole wheat pasta, wild rice, quinoa.

Breads and crackers: 100 percent whole grain European-style crackers, whole grain bread (2 to 3 grams fiber per 80 calories), whole wheat tortillas, whole wheat English muffins.

Beverages

Plain or sparkling water; seltzer; club soda; black, green, or herbal tea; kombucha; black coffee (regular or decaf); yerba mate.

Condiments, Dressings, Spices, and Sweeteners

Condiments: Balsamic vinegar, red wine vinegar, rice vinegar, hot sauce, dill relish, salsa, picante sauce, dill pickles, sweet pickles, ketchup, mustard (yellow, Dijon, stone ground, and spicy brown), low-sugar BBQ sauce, low-fat mayonnaise, tofu-based mayonnaise, pickled ginger, wasabi paste, all-fruit jam.

Dressings: Reduced-fat balsamic or red wine vinaigrette, fat-free or light Italian, light Honey Dijon, lemon or lime juice, tahini-based.

Spices and seasonings: Spice blends (sodium-free), fresh garlic, fresh ginger, garlic powder, vanilla extract, salt, Bragg Liquid Aminos or reduced-sodium tamari sauce, ground cumin, low-sodium soy sauce, black pepper, cinnamon, oregano, bay leaves, basil, cayenne, cinnamon, cardamom, curry, paprika, nutmeg, rosemary, sea salt.

Sweeteners: Agave nectar, honey, maple syrup (look for grade B), brown rice syrup, turbinado sugar, stevia.

Fats, Oils, and Cooking Sprays

Extra-virgin olive oil, light olive oil, canola oil, sesame oil, grape seed oil, virgin coconut oil, olive oil cooking spray, canola oil cooking spray, organic butter.

Nuts, Seeds, and Nut and Seed Butters

Almonds, Brazil nuts, cashews, macadamia nuts, mixed nuts (unsalted), peanuts, pecans, pistachios, walnuts, flaxseeds, pumpkin seeds, sunflower seeds, sesame seeds, peanut butter (natural, unsalted), almond butter (natural, unsalted), cashew butter, tahini (sesame seed butter), sunflower seed butter.

Frozen Foods

Vegetables: Cauliflower, green beans, broccoli, spinach, mixed vegetables, collards, corn, carrots, peas, peppers.

Fruit: Raspberries, blueberries, strawberries, mangoes, bananas, pineapple, fruit juice bars.

Protein: Fish fillets (salmon, cod, tilapia, or tuna), chicken breasts, lean beef, bison burgers, shrimp, vegetarian burgers.

Canned Foods

Beans, tomatoes, corn, tuna, pineapple, peaches in juice, fruit cocktail in juice, peas (no salt added), mixed vegetables (no salt added), sweet corn (no salt added), green beans (no salt added), sardines, wild salmon, olives, artichoke hearts, and coconut milk.

Appliances and Kitchen Tools
Essential

Blender, cutting boards, sharp knives (8- or 10-inch chef's knife, paring knife, and bread knife), peeler, measuring cups, measuring spoons, digital food or postal scale, pots and pans, salad spinner, toaster, handheld citrus juicer, colander, food processor, wooden spoons, spatula, rubber spatula, ladle, can opener, kitchen timer.

Helpful and Inexpensive

Nut chopper, steamer, wire mesh strainer, pepper mill, apple corer, slotted metal spoons, tongs, citrus squeezer.

Helpful and More Costly

Electric kettle, griddle, waffle iron, pressure cooker, rice cooker, Vitamix, Champion juicer, slow cooker, bread machine, vacuum-seal food saver, food dehydrator, toaster oven, coffee grinder (for flaxseed and spices).

CHAPTER 20

Coach Yourself Thin Meal Plans

Meal Planner: Breakfast Ideas

Look for the column that matches your CYT Calorie Level for specific portion guidance. See www.novowellness.com for more menu ideas.

		CYT 1,100–1,400	CYT 1,500–1,700
BREAKFAST #1	**Egg White Omelet** Egg White Omelet with onions, mushrooms, and bell pepper 100% whole grain toast Butter or all-fruit jam Raspberries Cup tea or coffee **Egg White Omelet:** Lightly coat a small skillet with cooking spray and place it over medium heat. Add the egg whites or egg substitute, onion, mushroom, and bell pepper. As the mixture sets, lift the edges, letting the uncooked portion flow underneath. When the eggs are set, fold the omelet in half.	(230 calories) Egg White Omelet: whites from 3 large eggs (or ½ cup egg substitute) and 2 Tbsp each chopped onions, mushrooms, and bell pepper 1 slice whole grain toast 1 cup raspberries *Choose one:* • 1 pat butter • 1 Tbsp jam • Half-and-half and/or sugar to total about 40 calories in tea or coffee (1 Tbsp half-and-half = 20 calories, 1 tsp sugar = 16 calories) Cup tea or coffee	(280 calories) Egg White Omelet: whites from 6 large eggs (or ¾ cup egg substitute) and 2 Tbsp each chopped onions, mushrooms, and bell pepper 1 slice whole grain toast 1 cup raspberries *Choose one:* • 1 pat butter • 1 Tbsp jam • Half-and-half and/or sugar to total about 40 calories in tea or coffee (1 Tbsp half-and-half = 20 calories, 1 tsp sugar = 16 calories) Cup tea or coffee

CYT 1,800–2,100	CYT 2,200–2,400	CYT 2,500
(360 calories)	(420 calories)	(460 calories)
Egg White Omelet: whites from 6 large eggs (or ¾ cup egg substitute) and 2 Tbsp each chopped onions, mushrooms, and bell pepper	Egg White Omelet: whites from 6 large eggs (or ¾ cup egg substitute) and 2 Tbsp each chopped onions, mushrooms, and bell pepper	Egg White Omelet: whites from 6 large eggs (or ¾ cup egg substitute) and 2 Tbsp each chopped onions, mushrooms, and bell pepper
2 slices whole grain toast	2 slices whole grain toast	2 slices whole grain toast
1 cup raspberries	1 cup raspberries	1 cup raspberries
Choose one:	1 pat butter or 1 Tbsp jam	2 pats butter or 2 Tbsp jam
• 1 pat butter	Half-and-half and/or sugar to total about 40 calories in tea or coffee (1 Tbsp half-and-half = 20 calories, 1 tsp sugar = 16 calories)	Half-and-half and/or sugar to total about 40 calories in tea or coffee (1 Tbsp half-and-half = 20 calories, 1 tsp sugar = 16 calories)
• 1 Tbsp jam		
• Half-and-half and/or sugar to total about 40 calories in tea or coffee (1 Tbsp half-and-half = 20 calories, 1 tsp sugar = 16 calories)	Cup tea or coffee	Cup tea or coffee
Cup tea or coffee		

Meal Planner: Breakfast Ideas (cont.)

		CYT 1,100–1,400	CYT 1,500–1,700
BREAKFAST #2	**Oatmeal & Cottage Cheese** Oatmeal Soy, almond, rice, or skim milk Nonfat cottage cheese Peaches Tea or coffee Follow the directions on the oatmeal package.	(230 calories) ½ cup oatmeal, cooked 1 tsp brown sugar ½ cup milk ¼ cup nonfat cottage cheese 2 canned peach halves or 1 fresh peach, sliced Cup tea or coffee	(280 calories) ½ cup oatmeal, cooked 1 tsp raisins 1 tsp brown sugar *Choose one:* • ½ cup milk and ¼ cup nonfat cottage cheese • ½ cup nonfat cottage cheese 2 canned peach halves or 1 fresh peach, sliced Cup tea or coffee
BREAKFAST #3	**ProBerry Protein Shake** Almonds Medjool date Water Blueberries Protein powder Banana, frozen Ice (optional) **ProBerry Protein Shake:** Blend almonds, pitted date, and water thoroughly for two minutes. Add blueberries and protein powder and blend for another 30 seconds. Add frozen slices of banana and blend until smooth.	(230 calories) 7 almonds 1 Medjool date 1 cup water ¼ cup blueberries ½ scoop whey protein powder (45 calories and 10 grams of protein) ½ medium to large banana, frozen, sliced Ice if desired to make shake thicker	(280 calories) 9 almonds 1 Medjool date 1 cup water ¼ cup blueberries ½ scoop whey protein powder (45 calories and 10 grams of protein) 1 medium to large banana, frozen, sliced Ice if desired to make shake thicker

CYT 1,800–2,100	CYT 2,200–2,400	CYT 2,500
(360 calories)	(420 calories)	(460 calories)
1 cup oatmeal, cooked	1 cup oatmeal, cooked	1 cup oatmeal, cooked
1 tsp raisins	1 Tbsp raisins	1 Tbsp raisins
1 tsp brown sugar	1 tsp brown sugar	1 tsp brown sugar
Choose one:	½ cup milk	½ cup milk
• ½ cup milk and ¼ cup nonfat cottage cheese	½ cup nonfat cottage cheese	¾ cup nonfat cottage cheese
• ½ cup nonfat cottage cheese	2 canned peach halves or 1 fresh peach, sliced	2 canned peach halves or 1 fresh peach, sliced
2 canned peach halves or 1 fresh peach, sliced	Cup tea or coffee	Half-and-half and/or sugar to total about 40 calories in tea or coffee (1 Tbsp half-and-half = 20 calories, 1 tsp sugar = 16 calories)
Cup tea or coffee		Cup tea or coffee
(360 calories)	(420 calories)	(460 calories)
9 almonds	15 almonds	15 almonds
1 Medjool date	1 Medjool date	1 Medjool date
1 cup water	1 cup water	1 cup water
½ cup blueberries	⅔ cup blueberries	⅔ cup blueberries
1 scoop whey protein powder (90 calories and 20 grams of protein)	1 scoop whey protein powder (90 calories and 20 grams of protein)	1 scoop whey protein powder (90 calories and 20 grams of protein)
1 large banana, frozen, sliced	1 large banana, frozen, sliced	2 medium bananas, frozen, sliced
Ice if desired to make shake thicker	Ice if desired to make shake thicker	Ice if desired to make shake thicker

Meal Planner: Lunch Ideas

Look for the column that matches your CYT Calorie Level for specific portion guidance. See www.novowellness.com for more menu ideas.

	CYT 1,100–1,400	CYT 1,500–1,800
Rotisserie Chicken Takeout	**CYT 1,100–1,300** (270 calories)	**CYT 1,500 –1,800** (440 calories)
Chicken breast, thighs, or drumstick	3 oz chicken (without skin)	4 oz chicken (without skin)
Sweet potato (see note below)	3 oz sweet potato (¼ large)	6 oz sweet potato (½ large)
Mixed vegetables (see note below)	1 cup mixed vegetables with balsamic vinegar, salt, and pepper	1 cup mixed vegetables with balsamic vinegar, salt, and pepper
Balsamic vinegar		1 tsp oil or butter for the vegetables
Salt	**CYT 1,400** (400 calories)	
Pepper		
Sweet potato: Bake at 400°F for 45 minutes or until soft when poked with a fork.	4 oz chicken (without skin)	
Vegetables: Put 1 inch of water in a saucepan and add the vegetables (with or without a steamer). Cover and cook over medium heat for 8 to 10 minutes, or until the vegetables are the desired tenderness.	6 oz sweet potato (½ large) 1 cup mixed vegetables with balsamic vinegar, salt, and pepper	

LUNCH #1

CYT 1,900–2,100	CYT 2,200–2,400	CYT 2,500
CYT 1,900 (500 calories)	**CYT 2,200** (630 calories)	**CYT 2,500** (750 calories)
4 oz chicken (without skin)	5 oz chicken (without skin)	5 oz chicken (without skin)
6 oz sweet potato (½ large)	6 oz sweet potato (½ large)	9 oz sweet potato (¾ large)
1 cup mixed vegetables with balsamic vinegar, salt, and pepper	1 cup mixed vegetables with balsamic vinegar, salt, and pepper	1 cup mixed vegetables with balsamic vinegar, salt, and pepper
1 tsp oil or butter for the vegetables	2 tsp oil or butter for the vegetables	1 Tbsp oil or butter for the vegetables
Small apple or other fruit serving (see list on page 151)	Small apple or other fruit serving (see list on page 151)	Small apple or other fruit serving (see list on page 151)
CYT 2,000–2,100 (580 calories)	**CYT 2,300–2,400** (670 calories)	
5 oz chicken	6 oz chicken (without skin)	
6 oz sweet potato (½ large)	6 oz sweet potato (½ large)	
1 cup mixed vegetables with balsamic vinegar, salt, and pepper	1 cup mixed vegetables with balsamic vinegar, salt, and pepper	
2 tsp oil or butter for the vegetables	2 tsp oil or butter for the vegetables	
Small apple or other fruit serving (see list on page 151)	Small apple or other fruit serving (see list on page 151)	

Meal Planner: Lunch Ideas (cont.)

	CYT 1,100–1,400	CYT 1,500–1,900	
Veggie Burger & Garden Salad Veggie burger on whole wheat bun Mustard, ketchup, and dill pickles Garden Salad Salad dressing **Garden Salad:** Combine 2 cups mixed greens; 1 small carrot, sliced; ½ cup cucumber slices; and 2 tomato slices	**CYT 1,000–1,300** (270 calories) Veggie burger (120 calories) on ½ whole wheat bun 2 tsp mustard 1 Tbsp ketchup 3 dill pickle slices 2 cups Garden Salad 1 Tbsp light salad dressing (60 calories) **CYT 1,400** (400 calories) Veggie burger (120 calories) on whole wheat bun 2 tsp mustard 1 Tbsp ketchup 3 dill pickle slices 2 cups Garden Salad 1 Tbsp salad dressing (60 calories) 1 fruit serving (see list on page 151)	**CYT 1,500–1,800** (440 calories) Veggie burger (120 calories) on whole wheat bun 2 tsp mustard 1 Tbsp ketchup 3 dill pickle slices 2 cups Garden Salad 1 Tbsp salad dressing (60 calories) 1 fruit serving (see list on page 151) **CYT 1,900** (500 calories) Veggie burger (120 calories) on whole wheat bun 2 tsp mustard 1 Tbsp ketchup 3 dill pickle slices 2 cups Garden Salad 1 Tbsp salad dressing (60 calories) 1 fruit serving (see list on page 151) *Choose one:* • Multigrain pretzels (80 calories) • Baked corn chips (80 calories) • ½ low-fat granola bar (80 calories)	

LUNCH #2

CYT 2,000–2,100	CYT 2,200–2,400	CYT 2,500

CYT 2,000–2,100
(580 calories)

Veggie burger (120 calories) on whole wheat bun

2 tsp mustard

1 Tbsp ketchup

3 dill pickle slices

2 cups Garden Salad

1 Tbsp salad dressing (60 calories)

1 fruit serving (see list on page 151)

Choose one:

- 1 oz multigrain pretzels (140 calories)

- 1 oz baked corn chips (140 calories)

- 1 low-fat granola bar (140 calories)

CYT 2,200 (630 calories)

Veggie burger (120 calories) on whole wheat bun

2 tsp mustard

1 Tbsp ketchup

3 dill pickle slices

2 cups Garden Salad

2 Tbsp salad dressing (100 calories)

1 fruit serving (see list on page 151)

Choose one:

- 1 oz multigrain pretzels (140 calories)

- 1 oz baked corn chips (140 calories)

- 1 low-fat granola bar (140 calories)

CYT 2,300–2,400
(670 calories)

Veggie burger (120 calories) on whole wheat bun

Slice of low-fat American cheese (40 calories)

2 tsp mustard

1 Tbsp ketchup

3 dill pickle slices

2 cups Garden Salad

2 Tbsp salad dressing (100 calories)

1 fruit serving (see list on page 151)

Choose one:

- 1 oz multigrain pretzels (140 calories)

- 1 oz baked corn chips (140 calories)

- 1 low-fat granola bar (140 calories)

CYT 2,500 (750 calories)

Veggie burger (120 calories) on whole wheat bun

Slice of American cheese (80 calories)

2 tsp mustard

1 Tbsp ketchup

3 dill pickle slices

2 cups Garden Salad

2 Tbsp salad dressing (100 calories)

1 fruit serving (see list on page 151)

Choose one:

- 1 oz multigrain pretzels (140 calories)

- 1 oz baked corn chips (140 calories)

- 1 low-fat granola bar (140 calories)

		CYT 1,100–1,400	CYT 1,500–1,800	
LUNCH #3	**Higher Protein Garden Salad** Garden Salad with chicken breast, turkey breast, roast beef, smoked salmon, or tempeh* **Garden Salad:** Combine 4 cups mixed greens; 1 medium carrot, sliced; 1 cup cucumber slices; and 2 tomato slices. Add your choice of protein. *You can substitute any of the following for 1 ounce of protein in your salad: ¼ cup nonfat cottage cheese 1 hard-boiled egg ½ cup green peas ¼ cup edamame or other bean	**CYT 1,100–1,300** (270 calories) Garden Salad 3 oz protein 1–2 Tbsp salad dressing (60 calories) **CYT 1,400** (400 calories) Garden Salad 3 oz protein Choose one: Additional 1 oz protein 1 Tbsp salad dressing (60 calories) Whole grain crackers (80 calories; see label)	**CYT 1,500–1,800** (440 calories) Garden Salad 4 oz protein 1–2 Tbsp salad dressing (80 calories) Whole grain crackers (80 calories; see label)	

CYT 1,900–2,100	CYT 2,200–2,400	CYT 2,500
CYT 1,900 (500 calories)	**CYT 2,200** (630 calories)	**CYT 2,500** (750 calories)
Garden Salad	Garden Salad	Garden Salad
5 oz protein	6 oz protein	6 oz protein
1–2 Tbsp salad dressing (60 calories)	2 Tbsp salad dressing (80 calories)	2 Tbsp salad dressing (80 calories)
Whole grain crackers (120 calories; see label)	Whole grain crackers (140 calories; see label)	2 slices avocado
		5 medium olives
CYT 2,000–2,100 (580 calories)	**CYT 2,300–2,400** (670 calories)	Whole grain crackers (160 calories; see label)
Garden Salad	Garden Salad	Apple or other fruit (see list on page 151)
6 oz protein	6 oz protein	
2 Tbsp salad dressing (80 calories)	2 Tbsp salad dressing (80 calories)	
Whole grain crackers (140 calories; see label)	Whole grain crackers (140 calories; see label)	
	Apple or other fruit (see list on page 151)	

Meal Planner: Dinner Ideas

Look for the column that matches your CYT Calorie Level for specific portion guidance. See www.novowellness.com for more menu ideas.

	CYT 1,100–1,500	CYT 1,600–1,900
Grilled Chicken, Basmati Rice, and Broccoli Grilled chicken breast BBQ sauce or other sauce Basmati rice Butter or olive oil Broccoli with lemon or balsamic vinegar **Rice:** Follow the directions on the rice package or bring 2 cups water and 1 cup rice to a boil. Reduce the heat after 1 minute, cover, and simmer until completely cooked (10 to 15 minutes for white rice and 30 to 40 minutes for brown rice).	**CYT 1,100–1,200** (400 calories) 4 oz grilled chicken breast 2 Tbsp BBQ or other sauce (25 calories) ½ cup basmati rice, cooked 1 tsp butter or olive oil 1 cup steamed broccoli with lemon or balsamic vinegar **CYT 1,300–1,500** (490 calories) 4 oz grilled chicken breast 2 Tbsp BBQ or other sauce (25 calories) 1 cup basmati rice, cooked 1 tsp butter or olive oil 1 cup steamed broccoli with lemon or balsamic vinegar	**CYT 1,600–1,800** (570 calories) 4 oz grilled chicken breast 2 Tbsp BBQ or other sauce (25 calories) 1 cup basmati rice, cooked 1 tsp butter or olive oil 1 cup steamed broccoli with lemon or balsamic vinegar 1 whole grain dinner roll **CYT 1,900** (610 calories) 4 oz grilled chicken breast 2 Tbsp BBQ sauce or other sauce (25 calories) 1 cup basmati rice, cooked 2 tsp butter or olive oil 1 cup steamed broccoli with lemon or balsamic vinegar 1 whole grain dinner roll

DINNER #1

CYT 2,000–2,200	CYT 2,300	CYT 2,400–2,500
CYT 2,000 (660 calories) 5 oz grilled chicken breast 2 Tbsp BBQ or other sauce (25 calories) 1 cup basmati rice, cooked 1 Tbsp butter or olive oil 1 cup steamed broccoli with lemon or balsamic vinegar 1 whole grain dinner roll	**CYT 2,300** (840 calories) 6 oz grilled chicken breast 2 Tbsp BBQ or other sauce (25 calories) 1½ cups basmati rice, cooked 1 Tbsp butter or olive oil 1 cup steamed broccoli with lemon or balsamic vinegar 1 whole grain dinner roll	**CYT 2,400–2,500** (910 calories) 7 oz grilled chicken breast 2 Tbsp BBQ or other sauce (25 calories) 1½ cups basmati rice, cooked 1 Tbsp butter or olive oil 1 cup steamed broccoli with lemon or balsamic vinegar 1 whole grain dinner roll
CYT 2,100–2,200 (740 calories) 5 oz grilled chicken breast 2 Tbsp BBQ or other sauce (25 calories) 1½ cups basmati rice, cooked 2 tsp butter or olive oil 1 cup steamed broccoli with lemon or balsamic vinegar 1 whole grain dinner roll		

		CYT 1,100–1,500	CYT 1,600–1,900
DINNER #2	**Sub Sandwich with Marinated Veggies** Whole grain sub roll Turkey breast, chicken breast, lean ham (lower sodium), or other sliced meat Lettuce Tomato Onion Dill pickle Mustard or low-fat mayonnaise **Summer Cucumber Salad** Makes 2 cups 1 large red, yellow, or orange bell pepper, cored and chopped 1 large cucumber, peeled and chopped ¼ cup chopped red onion ½ teaspoon dried dill 2 tablespoons balsamic vinegar 2 tablespoons Bragg Liquid Aminos or reduced-sodium tamari sauce ¼ teaspoon black pepper In a mixing bowl, combine the bell pepper, cucumber, onion, dill, vinegar, liquid aminos or tamari, and black pepper. Toss to combine and refrigerate for at least 2 hours for best flavor. Store refrigerated in a sealed container. It will keep for up to 5 days.	**CYT 1,100–1,200** (400 calories) 2 oz sub roll (160 calories) 3 oz chicken breast, turkey breast, or ham (150 calories) Lettuce, as desired 2 slices tomato 1 slice onion 2 slices dill pickle 2 tsp mustard or 1 Tbsp low-fat mayonnaise (35 calories) ½ cup Summer Cucumber Salad	**CYT 1,600–1,800** (570 calories) 3 oz sub roll (240 calories) 4 oz chicken breast, turkey breast, or ham (200 calories) Lettuce, as desired 2 slices tomato 1 slice onion 2 slices dill pickle 2 tsp mustard or 2 Tbsp low-fat mayonnaise (70 calories) 1 cup Summer Cucumber Salad
		CYT 1,300–1,500 (490 calories) 2 oz sub roll (160 calories) 4 oz chicken breast, turkey breast, or ham (200 calories) Lettuce, as desired 2 slices tomato 1 slice onion 2 slices dill pickle 2 tsp mustard or 2 Tbsp low-fat mayonnaise (70 calories) 1 cup Summer Cucumber Salad	**CYT 1,900** (610 calories) 3 oz sub roll (240 calories) 4 oz chicken breast, turkey breast, or ham (200 calories) Lettuce, as desired 2 slices tomato 1 slice onion 2 slices dill pickle 2 tsp mustard or 2 Tbsp low-fat mayonnaise (70 calories) 1 cup Summer Cucumber Salad with 1 tsp olive oil as dressing

CYT 2,000–2,200	CYT 2,300	CYT 2,400–2,500
CYT 2,000 (660 calories)	**CYT 2,300** (840 calories)	**CYT 2,400–2,500** (910 calories)
3 oz sub roll (240 calories)	4 oz sub roll (320 calories)	4 oz sub roll (320 calories)
5 oz chicken breast, turkey breast, or ham (250 calories)	6 oz chicken breast, turkey breast, or ham (250 calories)	6 oz chicken breast, turkey breast, or ham (200 calories)
Lettuce, as desired	Lettuce, as desired	Lettuce, as desired
2 slices tomato	2 slices tomato	2 slices tomato
1 slice onion	1 slice onion	1 slice onion
2 slices dill pickle	2 slices dill pickle	2 slices dill pickle
2 tsp mustard or 2 Tbsp low-fat mayonnaise (70 calories)	2 tsp mustard or 2 Tbsp low-fat mayonnaise (70 calories)	2 tsp mustard or 2 Tbsp low-fat mayonnaise (70 calories)
1 cup Summer Cucumber Salad with 1 tsp olive oil as marinade	1 cup Summer Cucumber Salad with 1 tsp olive oil as dressing	1½ cups Summer Cucumber Salad with 2 tsp olive oil as dressing
CYT 2,100–2,200 (740 calories)		
4 oz sub roll (320 calories)		
4 oz chicken breast, turkey breast, or ham (200 calories)		
Lettuce, as desired		
2 slices tomato		
1 slice onion		
2 slices dill pickle		
2 tsp mustard or 2 Tbsp low-fat mayonnaise (70 calories)		
1 cup Summer Cucumber Salad with 1 tsp olive oil as dressing		

	CYT 1,100–1,500	CYT 1,600–1,900
DINNER #3 **Restaurant Meal** Fish, chicken, or turkey Soup, broth-based Cooked vegetables or salad without meat, cheese, eggs, nuts, seeds, or croutons Coffee, tea, or sparkling water	**CYT 1,100–1,200** (400 calories) ½ grilled or baked fish, chicken, or turkey entrée Bowl of soup Side steamed vegetables or large salad Balsamic vinegar or lemon 1 bite any dessert (if desired) Cup tea, coffee, or sparkling water **CYT 1,300–1,500** (490 calories) ½ portion grilled or baked fish, chicken, or turkey entrée Bowl of soup Side steamed vegetables or large salad 1 Tbsp salad dressing 1 bite any dessert Cup tea, coffee, or sparkling water	**CYT 1,600–1,800** (570 calories) Grilled or baked fish, chicken, or turkey entrée Side steamed vegetables or large salad 1 Tbsp salad dressing (50 calories) 1 bite any dessert (if desired) Cup tea, coffee, or sparkling water **CYT 1,900** (610 calories) Grilled or baked fish, chicken, or turkey entrée Side steamed vegetables or large salad 2 Tbsp salad dressing (100 calories) 1 bite any dessert (if desired) Cup tea, coffee, or sparkling water

CYT 2,000–2,200	CYT 2,300	CYT 2,400–2,500
CYT 2,000 (660 calories) Grilled or baked fish, chicken, or turkey entrée Bowl of soup Side steamed vegetables or large salad 2 Tbsp salad dressing (100 calories) 1 bite any dessert (if desired) Cup tea, coffee, or sparkling water **CYT 2,100–2,200** (740 calories) Grilled or baked fish, chicken, or turkey entrée Bowl of soup Side steamed vegetables or large salad 2 Tbsp salad dressing (100 calories) Two bites any dessert (if desired) Cup tea, coffee, or sparkling water	**CYT 2,300** (840 calories) Grilled or baked fish, chicken, or turkey entrée Bowl of soup Side steamed vegetables or large salad 2 Tbsp salad dressing (100 calories) Two bites any dessert (if desired) Cup tea or coffee with milk and sugar (40 calories)	**CYT 2,400–2,500** (910 calories) Grilled or baked fish, chicken, or turkey entrée Bowl of soup Side of steamed vegetables or large salad 2 Tbsp salad dressing (100 calories) ½ dessert if desired (typical size slice of cake, pie, etc.) Cup tea, coffee, or sparkling water

PART 5

HEALTHY EXERCISE GUIDELINES

As we have mentioned previously, it is not our intention to outline a rigid exercise plan for you to follow to a T. One plan does not work for everyone. Therefore, rather than tell you exactly which exercises you should do to lose weight, our Healthy Exercise Guidelines are designed to provide a template for success: the basic fitness knowledge you need in order to choose the kinds of exercise that work for you and that you truly enjoy. This includes translating the common components of a fitness plan into easy-to-understand language and giving you the choice and the tools to either follow a very basic plan or to add more elements as your interest and ability increase.

> *Give a man a fish and you feed him for a day. Teach a man to fish and you feed him for a lifetime.*
>
> —Chinese Proverb

CHAPTER 21

Exercise Philosophy

There are four simple guidelines that we believe to be the basis of success with your exercise plan. We introduced them in "Regaining Your Balance" (page 57) and expound on them below. Keep them in mind as you learn about the components that follow. They will help you establish realistic expectations, discover a plan that works for you, and stay motivated.

FORM FOLLOWS FUNCTION (AND GENETICS)

You get out of your exercise what you put into it, and the more fit you are, the more it shows in the form of a leaner and better-functioning body. If your exercise plan consists of the same old activities week in and week out or, even worse, involves your quitting and starting over at the same level again and again, chances are that your fitness level isn't going to improve. The people we've worked with who've made transformations in their body composition have also made transformations in their fitness level. Over time, they have seen their ability to do physical work increase. They go faster or harder in their cardio workouts, complete more advanced exercise classes with less effort, and lift more weight in their strength training.

The key is to balance your expectations with your abilities, limitations, and motivation. (See "Expecting Greatness" on page 46 to review why it is important to have both realistic expectations and an expansive vision.)

It is also important to recognize that genetics play a role. They influence both how much you are able to improve your fitness level and how your body will look when you reach a high level of fitness. Comparing yourself to supermodels or professional athletes may feel motivating at first, but it is a trap. Eventually, the frustration caused by the difference in your results and the body shape and size of a model or athlete will undermine your resolve. It would be more fair to look at your family members, especially those that take care of their health, or even to compare yourself with how you looked at your most fit than it would be to look to a stranger for inspiration. But the best strategy of all is to stay focused on the powerful, beautiful, and vital person you become as your fitness level and shape change. Stick to comparing your results with where you began, and aim to increase the joy you get out of life, as well as improve the way you look.

KEEP IT SIMPLE

It's common to overcomplicate exercise, especially when you're first starting out. You might seek out the newest, most popular workout in an effort to speed up your weight loss, but end up slowing yourself down because the workout is too advanced for you. It's a classic example of trying to be the hare when, clearly, the tortoise will win the race.

Or you might get caught up in logistics: whether you should do strength training before cardio or the other way around; whether you should eat before you exercise or exercise on an empty stomach; whether you should exercise in the morning or the afternoon; whether you should perform intervals rather than run or walk at a steady pace. Worrying too much about these details makes exercise seem so mysterious that it holds you back from doing anything at all.

The truth is, neither the superhard workouts nor the finer points of training will matter one bit if you're not still exercising a month from now, and 6 months from now. It's like asking about how to navigate complicated investment tools before you've saved any money.

In the beginning, the difference between exercising one way and exercising another is not nearly as important as just getting out there and moving!

LISTEN TO YOUR BODY

It's a cliché, but it's still advice that most people forget to heed. If you experience pain in any joint during exercise, stop. Pain is a sign of an imbalance: Your muscles may be too tight or too weak to perform certain movements correctly and safely. At that point, the advice of your doctor or physical therapist takes precedence over any part of your exercise plan that exacerbates your symptoms. A professional can help you assess the physical imbalances or limitations that may be preventing normal, pain-free movement. It is wise to check with your doctor before beginning any exercise program, and make sure you continue to follow up as you progress with your lifestyle change.

As we mention earlier in this book, many people expect too much from their bodies in the beginning and yet cannot envision the great things their bodies could do if given the time. So they just push until their body breaks rather than allowing time to adapt and get stronger.

Why take what was not important yesterday and approach it with a "must do it or else" attitude today? You can't make up for years and years in one day. Lighten up and be patient. The urgency is a trap, and by rushing your progress, you're setting yourself up to fail. Consistency is much more important than how hard you push when you first start out.

MAKE IT FUN

One of the keys to sticking with exercise is to find something you enjoy and/or that gives you the strength and confidence to do the things you want to do in life. We have lost much of our sense of play in today's busy world. Going to the gym can seem like just one more task that has to be

---

When to Ask Questions about Your Exercise Plan

As long as you have no serious physical limitations, there is no reason that you cannot go for a simple walk, ride a bicycle, or take a dance class. However, if either your doctor's advice or an injury or physical pain limit or restrict your activity, don't be afraid to ask for help deciding what types of exercise are appropriate for you. And if you are attempting something completely new, ask for assistance in learning the proper technique. The advice of your doctor, physical therapist, personal trainer, or an experienced and attentive exercise class instructor is invaluable in these situations.

done. You can make your movement more fun by selecting activities that you feel are more like recreation or play: go to dance class, play a sport, get outside, or include your spouse or kids.

And if the activity itself isn't inherently fun, then try to link it to the ability to do something that is. Maybe lifting weights in the gym seems tedious. But by connecting the strength you gain at the gym to your ability to play with your children or grandchildren, you make the gym a slightly more desirable place to go.

Finally, there is evidence that exercising outdoors is good for your health. Exercising outside has been shown to have a greater effect on improving mood and decreasing anger, anxiety, and depression than the equivalent exercise performed indoors. That's not to say that indoor exercise is not recommended. Many people live in areas where exercising outdoors may be unsafe, and there are certain types of exercise, such as strength training with machines or dance-based aerobics, that are better done in a gym. But getting out to romp and play once in a while can give your exercise an added boost!

CHAPTER 22

Introduction to the Components of Fitness

An in-depth look at all of the components of fitness would require a whole separate book. (See the Resources on page 273 for recommendations.) What we will cover here are the basic parts of a well-rounded fitness program, as well as how you can use them to create a plan that works for you now and that teaches you how to adapt your plan to your changing needs as you progress on your weight-loss journey.

In the chapters that follow, we will introduce you to "activities of daily living," as well as what are generally considered to be the primary areas of fitness: cardio (aerobic or cardiovascular exercise) and strength training (resistance training). We will also discuss rejuvenation—the types of exercise that will help your muscles recover from your workouts and help you manage the cumulative physical and mental stresses of everyday life.

The chapters in this section each contain a short definition of each activity, what you can expect to gain, some basic information on what to do, and a suggested progression for getting the most out of your exercise. As you work through the progressions, keep the following guidelines in mind:

- Maintain a particular level for 2 to 3 weeks before moving to the next level.

- Feel free to move to a lower level if your energy, time constraints, or motivation demand it.

- Take an easy week that contains only recovery cardio, rejuvenation, and 2 or 3 complete rest days at least once every 3 months.

CHAPTER 23

Activities of Daily Living

Activities of daily living include noncontinuous activities and activities that are not metabolically demanding, such as those you might do during a normal day. "Noncontinuous" is open to interpretation. Our definition is any activity that takes less than 5 minutes to complete or that is interrupted by rest periods less than 5 minutes apart. And "not metabolically demanding" can vary from one person to another, but a good measuring stick is that this type of activity does not noticeably increase your breathing and heart rates. Gardening, housework, taking the stairs, walking to lunch, walking the dog, working in your yard, and bypassing those moving sidewalks at the airport are all good examples.

BENEFITS OF ACTIVITIES OF DAILY LIVING

Activities of daily living, or ADLs, are what make you a truly active person. If you are active, you don't just go to the gym for 30 minutes every day—you seize every opportunity to be active! The weight-loss benefit is that you burn more calories throughout your entire day, not just during the few hours per week that you do regular exercise. Reaching, bending, twisting, lifting, carrying, walking, and running are what we are built to do. If you take the time to fit more movement into your day, it will complement your regular exercise program and, we believe, give you a rewarding outlet for using the fitness you gain through exercise. If you can take the stairs without getting winded, then skipping the escalator will feel like a victory every time you do it!

HOW TO: ACTIVITIES OF DAILY LIVING

Wearing a pedometer to count the steps you take during both your daily activities and your formal workouts is a great way to track your daily movement. (Check the Resources on page 273 for guidance on what kind of pedometer to buy.) Put your pedometer on in the morning and count all the steps you have taken before you go to bed at night. Many people find that wearing a pedometer encourages them to be more active than they would be otherwise. If you participate in activities that do not register on the pedometer (such as cycling and swimming) and you want to include that exercise in your daily total, you can estimate 100 steps for each minute of exercise.

PROGRESSION FOR ACTIVITIES OF DAILY LIVING

Wear your pedometer all day for 2 weekdays and 1 weekend day to get an accurate picture of both workdays and days when your schedule is more flexible and varied. Average the steps taken on those 3 days and use this number as your baseline. Then work on increasing your weekly average by no more than 10 percent per week toward until you reach the "active" level.[1]

3,000–4,999 steps/day = sedentary

5,000–7,499 steps/day = lightly active

7,500–9,999 steps/day = moderately active

$\geq$10,000 steps/day = active

CHAPTER 24

Cardiovascular Exercise

Cardio is any form of movement that involves constantly working large muscle groups, significantly elevating your breathing and heart rates and keeping them elevated for as long as the movement is being performed. Cardio activities can be performed both outdoors and at the gym. They include:

Cross-country skiing	Stair-climbing
Cycling	Dance-based aerobics classes
Elliptical training	Swimming
Ice-skating or in-line skating	Walking or running
Indoor rowing	Water aerobics
Rowing	

Choose a cardio activity based on your level of conditioning and any physical limitations you have, including injuries, diseases, and joint pain. Also take into account whether you like to work out inside or outside and alone or in a group setting, as well as what facilities and resources you have easy access to.

BENEFITS OF CARDIO

Because cardio burns more calories in a shorter period of time than other common forms of exercise (such as resistance and flexibility training), it is often touted as the "best" exercise for people seeking to lose weight. While we don't believe that any "best" weight-loss exercise exists, cardio definitely does a great job of burning some serious calories and has a range of other physical benefits, including:

Improved endurance*

Reduced body fat

Reduced risk of cardiovascular disease

Prevention of non-insulin-dependent diabetes

Reduced blood pressure and/or risk of developing hypertension

Increase in HDL (good, protective) cholesterol

Reduced risk of stroke

Reduced risk of certain cancers, especially colon cancer in men and women and breast cancer in women

Reduced risk of osteoporosis

Lowered stress levels

Improved mood

Decreased risk of depression or reduced symptoms of depression

Decreased anxiety

*As your cardiovascular fitness improves, your circulatory and respiratory systems are better able to deliver oxygen-rich blood to your working muscles and your muscles are better able to use that oxygen to create energy.

HOW TO: CARDIO

According to the American College of Sports Medicine, adults need to participate in at least 150 minutes of moderate-intensity physical activity each week. This helps prevent weight gain and decreases the risk of chronic diseases associated with being overweight. A good way to look at this is that it equals 30 minutes of activity, 5 days per week. For better weight-loss results and maintenance, it is recommended that overweight and obese individuals perform 250 or more minutes of moderate-intensity physical activity each week.[1]

If you would like to cut down on your exercise time, you can get many of the same benefits by exercising at a higher intensity. (See page 194 to determine your intensity level.) For example, you could perform

60 to 75 minutes of vigorous activity per week as an alternative to 150 minutes of moderate activity.

Another way to measure your exercise is in calories burned. (The American College of Sports Medicine provides well-respected guidelines in its *Guidelines for Exercise Testing and Prescription*.) To lose weight, it is recommended that you build up to burning 300 to 500 calories per exercise session, or a total of 1,000 to 2,000 calories or more per week. The threshold of 1,000 calories is associated with improvements in health, while burning 2,000 calories or more per week is considered better for weight control.[2]

The problem is that measuring calorie burn is very difficult to do accurately. Charts and calculators can work well when the precise workload is known ("walking at 3.0 mph," for example). But for more general activities, such as aerobics, they might be far off the mark because there is no way to take into account the amount of work you do. Some cardio machines may estimate fairly closely, especially if they allow you to enter your body weight. But there is no way to know how close the numbers are to correct. Pedometers, heart rate monitors, and devices that use motion sensors track your movement do not "measure" calorie burn; they can only estimate it. If you do use a tool to estimate calorie burn, we recommend that you pick just one and stick with it to avoid comparing one result with another. And don't use the results to determine exactly how much you can eat and still lose weight. Instead, simply compare one workout to another and, over time, track how the number of calories burned per session increases.

Intensity

To help you zero in on how hard you are really working, use the information below to estimate your target heart rate and rate of perceived exertion (RPE).

Estimating Your Target Heart Rate

For guidance we again turn to recommendations provided by the American College of Sports Medicine.

1. Subtract your age from 220 to get your maximum heart rate (max HR).

Intensity versus Pace

Throughout this chapter, you will see references to "intensity" and "pace" when describing cardio exercise. In the context of our exercise plan, intensity refers to a particular heart rate or effort level and pace refers to how fast you move in order to reach a particular intensity level. For example, the pace you walk, run, cycle, or move in your aerobics class to bring your effort level to between 13 and 15 and your heart rate to 70 to 80 percent of your maximum is your "build" pace.

2. Calculate 55 and 90 percent of your max HR from step 1. This range should be your target HR (THR) to reach while engaging in cardio exercise. (See "Rating of Perceived Exertion," below, and "CYT Components of Cardio" on page 197 for more information on appropriate heart rate zones for different types of cardio workouts.)

3. During cardio exercise, place your first two fingers on one hand (don't use your thumb) side-by-side at the thumb side of your wrist on the other hand. Count for 20 seconds and multiply the number of beats by three—while still moving, if possible. This is your heart rate. For more accuracy, use a heart rate monitor. (See Resources on page 273 for information on how to shop for a good monitor.)[3]

Rating of Perceived Exertion (RPE)

One of the simplest and best ways to know if your workout is too easy, too hard, or just right is to tune in to how hard it feels to you. The tool for this is called the Rating of Perceived Exertion, or RPE.[4] The original scale was created by Swedish physiologist Gunnar Borg in 1982. Today, many variations of it are widely used in the fitness industry to help estimate intensity of exercise. Practice using the scale and you'll learn to trust what you feel. Remember: As a general rule, if it feels too hard, it is.

1 to 6 No exertion at all.

7 Very, very light: Extremely light movement. Like walking the aisles at the grocery store.

8

9 Very light: Like an easy stroll. You can hold a conversation without difficulty. (9 to 11 is appropriate for Recover workouts; see page 200.)

10

11 Light: A sense of moving with purpose, but still light enough that conversation is easy. (11 to 13 is appropriate for Comfort Zone and Sustain workouts; see page 198. RPE of 11 = heart rate of approximately 55 percent of max HR.)

12

13 Somewhat hard: Moderate intensity. You can talk in complete sentences, but your breathing is labored. (13 to 15 is appropriate for Build workouts; see page 198. RPE of 13 to 15 = heart rate range of approximately 70 to 80 percent of your max HR.)

14

15 Hard: Vigorous intensity. It takes focus to maintain your pace. Your breathing rate is elevated enough that talking is restricted to short phrases. (15 to 17 is appropriate for Speed workouts; see page 199. RPE of 15 to 17 = heart rate range of approximately 80 to 90 percent of your max HR.)

16

17 Very hard: Very vigorous intensity. Conversation is not possible. This pace cannot be maintained for more than a few minutes at a time.

18

19 Extremely hard: Near all-out to all-out exertion. This level is not recommended as a part of your regular exercise program.

20 Maximal

Note: If you take medications that alter your heart rate response to exercise, such as those for blood pressure and heart rhythm, you'll need to rely on RPE and not heart rate while doing cardio, unless your doctor prescribes a training heart rate specific to your current dose of medication.

CYT COMPONENTS OF CARDIO

Many people do the same cardio workout day in and day out, either keeping the intensity very light and watching TV or reading a book while they work out, or forcing their bodies to work at their limits every time they exercise. The first group of people are often frustrated by a lack of progress, while the second group tends to burn out or get injured very frequently.

The following four components of cardio workouts will help you break out of these common ruts. They are based on the concept of building up to a Comfort Zone workout and then modifying that workout by making it longer or harder to improve your fitness or easier to aid recovery. Your Comfort Zone workout is the duration and the intensity that you are able to do consistently, 3 to 6 days per week, without feeling that you are going too long, too hard, or too easy. Your comfortable duration will range from 30 minutes to an hour (see "Level 1" on page 200) and your intensity will range from light to moderate, or an RPE of 11 to 13 and/or a heart rate range of 55 to 70 percent of your maximum heart rate.

Guidelines and Example Workouts

The first step is to take a few weeks to establish your Comfort Zone workout. Start with an amount of cardio that feels achievable and comfortable to you. The exact amount will depend on your fitness level, but most people will fall somewhere between a lower end of 2 to 3 minutes and a higher end of 30 to 45 minutes to start.

To build up your Comfort Zone workout, each week you will increase the duration of your workout by:

1 to 2 minutes, if you begin with workouts of 10 minutes or less

2 to 3 minutes, if you begin with workouts of 11 to 20 minutes

3 to 5 minutes, if you begin with workouts of more than 20 minutes

Ideally, you will build up your Comfort Zone workout to 30 to 60 minutes. Choose the duration that feels right to you. And, as always, remember that it is far better to work out consistently in your Comfort Zone than to push too hard and get hurt or frustrated and quit!

Once your Comfort Zone workout is established, the duration does not change each week. (See Level 1 on page 200 for weekly guidelines and Tips on page 201 for instructions on changing your Comfort Zone.) However, you can add the following four components to your plan to take your fitness to the next level.

Sustain (Light to moderate intensity; RPE 11 to 13 and/or heart rate equal to 55 to 70 percent of your maximum heart rate): This is longer than your Comfort Zone workout but is performed at about the same intensity and is meant to build endurance.

This workout should be no more than 25 to 30 percent of your total weekly cardio minutes. For example, if you do 180 minutes per week, your Sustain workout can build up to 45 to 60 minutes.

Your Sustain workout should increase by no more than approximately 10 to 20 percent each week. The first time you increase your Sustain workout, apply the following guidelines to your Comfort Zone workout. Once you have established a new level for your Sustain workout, use the same guidelines but apply them to your current Sustain workout.

> Comfort Zone (only for initial increase) or current Sustain workout of < 30 minutes = increase Sustain workout by 3 to 5 minutes per week
>
> Comfort Zone (only for initial increase) or current Sustain workout of 30 to 60 minutes = increase Sustain workout by 5 to 10 minutes per week
>
> Comfort Zone (only for initial increase) or current Sustain workout of > 60 minutes = increase Sustain workout by 10 to 15 minutes per week

Build (Moderate to vigorous intensity; RPE 13 to 15 and/or heart rate equal to 70 to 80 percent of your maximum heart rate): Performed at just above the pace you can sustain comfortably in your Comfort Zone workout, Build workouts will increase your ability to sustain a higher level of work for a prolonged period.

The maximum number of minutes per week spent at Build pace should not exceed 10 to 20 percent of your total weekly cardio minutes. For example, if you do 180 minutes per week, you can do 18 to 36 minutes of Build work.

Workouts can be continuous, beginning with 10 minutes and building up to a maximum of 30 minutes. Increase your Build workouts by no more than 5 minutes per week and follow the guidelines above for maximum duration.

You can also maintain your Build pace for 5 to 15 minutes at a time, alternating with very short recoveries (easy walking) between each effort. Use a recovery of 1 minute for every 5 minutes at Build pace. (For example, 5 minutes at Build pace followed by 1 minute of recovery, 10 minutes at Build pace followed by 2 minutes of recovery, and so on.)

Begin with a total of no more than 15 total minutes per workout at Build pace and increase the total per workout by no more than 5 minutes each week, up to a maximum of 30 to 45 minutes per workout. You can divide up the time at Build pace however works best for you.

For example:

3 x 5 minutes, 1 x 10 minutes, 1 x 15 minutes = 15 minutes or less at Build pace

4 x 5 minutes, 2 x 15 minutes, 3 x 10 minutes, 1 x 15 minutes + 1 x 10 minutes = 20 to 30 minutes at Build pace

6 x 5 minutes, 3 x 15 minutes, 4 x 10 minutes, 2 x 15 minutes = 30 to 45 minutes at Build pace

Be sure to warm up at a light to moderate intensity for at least 5 minutes before beginning Build pace, and always cool down at a light intensity for at least 5 minutes after you finish your workout.

Speed (Vigorous intensity; RPE 15 to 17 and/or heart rate equal to 80 to 90 percent of your maximum heart rate): These are short bursts or intervals of much faster and harder cardio than you are able to maintain for a continuous workout. They're designed to build up your maximal cardiovascular fitness and the number of calories burned per exercise session.

The maximum number of minutes per week at Speed pace should not exceed 10 percent of your total weekly cardio minutes. For example, if you do 180 minutes per week, you can do up to 18 minutes of Speed work.

Speed workouts contain short intervals (1 to 5 minutes) of work at Speed pace, followed by a period of recovery that is anywhere from 50 to 100 percent as long as the preceding work interval. For example, if you do 2 minutes at Speed pace, it should be followed immediately by 1 to 2 minutes of recovery (easy walking). And if you do 5 minutes at Speed pace, it should be followed immediately by 2½ to 5 minutes of recovery.

You can divide up the time at Speed pace any way you like.

For example:

10 x 1 minute at Speed pace with a 1-minute recovery between each effort = 10 total minutes at Speed pace

4 x 3 minutes at Speed pace with a 1½-minute recovery between each effort = 12 total minutes at Speed pace

5 minutes at Speed pace with a 2½-minute recovery + 4 minutes at Speed pace with a 2-minute recovery + 3 minutes at Speed pace with a 1½-minute recovery + 2 minutes at Speed pace with a 1-minute recovery + 1 minute at Speed pace (then cool down) = 15 minutes at Speed pace

Be sure to warm up at a light to moderate intensity for at least 5 minutes before beginning Speed pace and cool down at a light intensity for at least 5 minutes after you finish your workout. Do not do two hard cardio workouts (Sustain, Build, or Speed) on consecutive days!

Recover (Very light intensity; RPE 10 or less and/or heart rate less than 55 percent of your maximum heart rate): This is shorter and easier than your Comfort Zone workout. These workouts should provide an "active recovery" from harder workouts. Do a Recover workout or complete rest days between your Sustain, Build, and Speed workouts.

PROGRESSION FOR CARDIO
Level 1 (Comfort Zone)

Build up to and maintain 150 to 300 minutes of moderate-intensity cardio per week by doing 30 to 60 minutes on 3 to 6 days per week. Do not significantly vary the intensity or duration of your workouts from day to day.

Level 2

Do 1 Sustain workout, 1 Recover workout, and 1 to 4 Comfort Zone workouts per week. Workout on a total of 3 to 6 days.

Level 3

Do 1 Build workout, 1 Sustain workout, 1 or 2 Recover workouts, and an optional 1 or 2 Comfort Zone workouts per week. Workout on a total of 3 to 6 days.

Level 4

Do 1 Speed workout, 1 Build workout, 1 Sustain workout, 1 or 2 Recover workouts, and an optional Comfort Zone workout per week. Workout on a total of 3 to 6 days.

Recovery Week

Do 2 or 3 Recover workouts and an optional 1 or 2 Comfort Zone workouts per week. Workout on a total of 2 to 5 days.

Tips

- Complete at least 3 to 4 weeks at one level before moving to the next level.
- Ideally, complete a Recovery week following 3 to 4 weeks of training at any of the above levels. At a maximum, complete 6 to 8 weeks at any of the above levels between Recovery weeks.
- Feel free to drop down to a previous level if you need a break from harder workouts. You could do this to take a mental and physical break from hard training or in response to a very busy period in your life (work deadlines, holidays, etc.).
- You can also drop back to Level 1 at any time to establish a new Comfort Zone workout. For example, if your Comfort Zone is 30 minutes and you feel ready to move that up to 45 minutes, simply use the guidelines above for increasing your Comfort Zone.

CHAPTER 25

Strength Training

Strength training is a great way to build up muscles and joints so they can better handle everyday tasks. It will give you the ability and confidence to stand up from a low chair, carry your groceries, lift a child, or climb stairs.

Strength training refers to exercising against some form of resistance to create muscular fatigue. It includes the use of:

Body weight (calisthenics)

Dumbbells (also known as free weights)

Kettlebells

Medicine balls

Resistance tubes or bands

Water resistance (using foam dumbbells, webbed gloves, etc.)

Machines of various types

While some group fitness classes and workout DVDs may incorporate weights, most of those workouts are not true strength training. They are typically a cross between strength and cardio, using light weights and a lot of reps to give you a high-intensity cardio workout. These workouts do help build muscle, in the same way that a Tour de France rider will strengthen his legs by riding, even though the activity is mostly cardio. But "true" strength training involves working the muscles to a significant level of fatigue in a short period of time against a relatively high (compared to cardio workouts) level of resistance. This workload helps you maintain or even build muscle. And more muscle means more calories burned, both at rest and during activity.

BENEFITS OF STRENGTH TRAINING

Strength training contributes to your weight-loss efforts by helping improve your mobility (which means that you'll burn more calories because you're willing and able to move more). It also helps prevent injuries that could disrupt your exercise by balancing your muscular strength (if you work all muscle groups), which improves your posture and helps you move more efficiently, and it keeps your joints protected and stabilized. Some other benefits include:

- Preservation of lean body mass as you age
- Reduced risk of cardiovascular disease
- Reduced risk of non-insulin-dependent diabetes
- Reduced blood pressure and/or risk of developing hypertension (though the effect has not proven to be as strong as with cardio training)
- Reduced risk of stroke
- Reduced risk of certain cancers, especially colon cancer in men and women and breast cancer in women
- Reduced risk of osteoporosis
- Lower incidence of lower back pain
- Decreased risk or reduced symptoms of depression

HOW TO: STRENGTH TRAINING

Below are the major variables that you can manipulate to add variety to and change the intensity of your strength workouts. There is no "perfect" strength workout or one that works best for weight loss. As long as you challenge yourself, include a lot of variety, and follow the guidelines below, you'll improve your fitness and greatly contribute to your weight-loss efforts.[1]

Difficulty

We define difficulty by how much balance, stabilization, and coordination is required to do a move correctly. Stabilization refers to the work your core (abdomen, lower back, and hips) does to help you maintain good form and posture during an exercise. For example, without proper stabilization, your back will move out of proper alignment during a heavy bench press and arch up off the bench. By increasing the difficulty of the exercises you're doing as your core fitness improves, you challenge and strengthen your core more thoroughly.

Low Difficulty: It is easier to perform a strength training exercise while you're lying on the floor or a bench or being supported by a machine. Also, moving in one plane at a time—forward and back (a squat), side to side (stepping to the left or right), or twisting (torso rotation)—is easier than moving in multiple planes at once. (See page 208 for specific examples of strength training exercises.)

High Difficulty: Less external stability makes strength training more difficult. Sitting on a stability ball while doing a strength training exercise is more difficult than sitting on a bench or chair. Standing exercises, especially those performed while standing on one foot or on a balance tool like a BOSU, are more difficult than sitting exercises. Moving in more than one plane, such as when you twist your torso to turn your shoulders while doing a squat, also increases difficulty.

Reps

A repetition, or rep, is one complete movement of an exercise from the starting position, through the full range of motion, and back to the starting position. A set (see "Sets" on page 206) is a group of repetitions. You'll gain the most strength by performing reps of an exercise until you reach muscular fatigue, or the point at which you cannot continue the movement with proper form. To allow the body to adapt to the new stresses of strength training, beginning exercisers will use a high number of reps (15 to 25) with lower resistance, while experienced exercisers are able to aim for fewer reps (8 to 12) with more challenging resistance. (See the following section for more information on resistance.)

Note: For body-weight exercises like pushups, lunges, and squats, you'll need to reverse this process. Start with a lower number of reps (8 to 12) and increase the number of reps (up to 25) as you get stronger.

Resistance

Use an amount of resistance that creates muscular fatigue within the rep ranges suggested above. You can increase resistance by changing the angle

Machines versus Natural Movements

It has long been asserted that beginning exercisers should use machines instead of free weights because they "guide" you through the movement and help you control the resistance safely. We believe, however, that more natural movements performed without the support of a chair back or chest pad, or those performed while standing or moving, are much more effective than exercises done while being fully supported and following the movement pattern that a machine dictates. This is because unsupported movements allow your body to move naturally and strengthen not just the primary muscles targeted by an exercise but also your core and other assisting muscles that provide stability for your spine and joints.

There are a few exceptions to this generalization. For example, machines used by physical therapists to help rehab people from injuries and muscle imbalances are essential to the isolation and strengthening of a particular muscle group.

Also, not all machines are created equal. For example, a chest or shoulder press machine can be riskier than free weights because it forces you into a "set" movement pattern that can harm your joints. A leg press machine, on the other hand, offers a good alternative for someone who lacks the ability to do a squat properly. Lat pulldown machines offer a good alternative to chinup exercises. A cable machine offers a myriad of ways to do exercises while standing up without any support at all, which makes it nearly identical to free weights.

Many people use machines when they begin resistance training because they feel that machines are less intimidating than free weights. We fully support your breaking into strength training with machines, but we do recommend that you use the suggested exercises in this chapter, as well as the resources we provide (see page 273), to learn other ways of performing your strength exercises.

of the movement, such as by doing pushups from your toes instead of your knees, squatting deeper, or using heavier dumbbells, stronger exercise tubing, or a heavier weight on a machine with a weight stack. If you cannot complete the target reps with good form, decrease the resistance during your next set or next exercise session. On the other hand, if you can do more than the target reps, increase the resistance or do a more difficult version of the exercise with less stabilization during your next set or exercise session (see "Difficulty" on page 203).

Do not try to use one weight for every exercise. If you attempt a lateral raise and then a dumbbell bench press with the same weight, you'll instantly realize that the lateral raise is far more difficult. When it comes to choosing resistance, evaluate each exercise separately.

Sets

As we mentioned earlier, reps of strength training exercises make up sets, and our recommended ranges for total sets per workout session are below. They are based on what will allow you to exercise each major strength training component—Stabilize, Push, Pull, and Move (see "CYT Components of Strength Training" on the opposite page)—in a reasonable amount of time.

To begin: Total of 5 to 10 sets. We recommend that you choose at least 1 Push, Pull, and Move exercise and at least 2 Core exercises. Perform 1 or 2 sets of each exercise.

More advanced: Total of 20 to 30 sets. We recommend that you choose at least 2 Push, Pull, and Move exercises and at least 3 Core exercises. Perform 2 or 3 sets of each exercise.

Rest between Sets

How long you should rest between sets depends entirely on what kind of strength training routine you're performing. Circuit workouts are designed to be performed by moving quickly from one exercise to another, typically using lighter resistance. In circuit training, you rest for 0 to 30 seconds between sets. In noncircuit workouts using heavier resistance, rest for 1 to 2 minutes between sets.

Speed of Movement

Slower lifting speeds are beneficial when you're learning a new movement because they allow your body to adapt to resistance training before you add the stress of moving quickly. Moving slowly also lets you learn how to properly stabilize your body and maintain good posture while lifting. Performing movements slowly means taking 2 seconds or longer to lift or move the resistance and 4 seconds or longer to return to the starting position.

Once you are used to the demands of strength training, you can increase your lifting speed. A moderate speed that is excellent for improving strength is 1 to 2 seconds to lift or move the resistance and 1 to 2 seconds to return to the starting position.

Very high speeds are associated with throwing and jumping exercises; these, by nature, require moving "as fast as possible." These types of exercises are performed in many fitness classes that involve jumping over hurdles, using kettlebells, or throwing medicine balls. Make sure that you've built up to the demands of such a class by getting used to more moderate lifting speeds first.

Frequency

For most fitness goals, working the whole body in one workout and performing that workout on 2 or 3 days per week is sufficient. More experienced exercisers can exercise 4 to 6 days per week by breaking a total body workout up into workouts for separate body parts, thus increasing the volume of exercise for each body part.

No matter how often you train, you can help prevent burnout and injury by not working the same body parts on consecutive days, allowing your body to recover properly from your strength workouts.

CYT COMPONENTS OF STRENGTH TRAINING

In the cardio section of this book, we focused on the *types* of workouts to include in a well-rounded program. But there are so many varieties of strength workouts—circuits, boot camp–type workouts, single sets of each exercise, multiple sets of each exercise, slow movements, fast movements, exercises that work one muscle group, exercises that work multiple muscle groups, and so on—that it would simply be impossible to recommend one over another. Despite what you will hear in the media, there is no "right" way to strength train to enhance weight loss. Variety is the real key. We recommend using a range of equipment (refer to page 202 for specifics) and a range of different exercises to make sure that your body is constantly challenged and to keep your motivation high.

The CYT Components of Strength Training that follow are the four key types of movement that we believe are essential to an effective workout. Whether you attend an exercise class, watch a DVD, or design your own workout, incorporating these moves into your weekly strength routine and following the guidelines in "How To: Strength Training" (see page 203) will guarantee that you're getting a well-rounded, total body workout.

There are literally thousands of strength training exercises available, and we do refer to some of these exercises to illustrate certain points and as examples of the four components of strength training. If you are unfamiliar with any of these exercises, you can find great photographs and even video examples by plugging any of the exercise names into an Internet search engine, or you can check the Resources section (see page 273) for reputable sources for viewing the exercises.

Ideally, you will use the information in this section to create a workout that works for you and that can be changed in infinite ways.

Components

Stabilize: The primary role of your core—your abdomen, lower back, and hips—is to stabilize your body. To get an idea of what stabilization feels like, hold both hands straight out in front of your chest and clasp your fingers together. Now ask a friend to push your hands up and down and side to side in an unpredictable pattern. Your ability to remain standing without losing your balance comes from the contraction of your core muscles as they resist your friend's pushing. That same contraction happens when you lift a suitcase, carry a laundry basket, or open a door. When it comes to strength training exercises, doing an abdominal crunch works your core, but not in the most valuable way. Because you lie on a stable surface (the floor) during a crunch, your core is reduced to flexing your spine, which is what happens as your head and shoulders lift from the floor, instead the harder job of keeping your body stable.

Examples of Stabilize exercises include (in order of ascending difficulty):

Supine hip bridge

Bicycle crunch

Prone plank

Alternating leg lift plank

Cable wood chop (*Note:* When integrated with squats, this is a Move exercise.)

Push and Pull: These are the two major types of moves performed by the upper body (the chest, back, arms, and shoulders).

Push refers to any upper body exercise that involves pushing resistance away from your body. These moves primarily use the muscles of your chest, the fronts of your shoulders, and your triceps. In everyday life, the resistance can come from a stationary object that you push against (such as pushing yourself up from the floor) or a mobile object that you push away (such as a baby stroller or a lawn mower).

Examples of Push exercises include (in order of ascending difficulty):

Dumbbell bench press

Cable chest press

Wall pushup

Standing cable chest press

Side plank pushup

Pull refers to any upper body exercise that involves pulling resistance toward your body. These moves primarily use the muscles of your back, the backs of your shoulders, and your biceps. In everyday life, the resistance can come from a stationary object that you pull against (such as a dog's leash when he tries to run away) or an object that you move toward your body (such as grocery bags out of your trunk or a door that you pull open).

Examples of Pull exercises include (in order of ascending difficulty):

Seated row machine

Lat pulldown (*Note:* Pull to the front of your body, not behind your head.)

One-arm dumbbell row

Standing cable row

Rotational row

Move: Any movement that works your entire lower body, from your hips to your toes. We chose this verb to remind you that the ultimate objective of lower body exercises is to improve your mobility. Your legs take you across a room, move you up the stairs, stand you up from a sitting position, and provide the base on which you lift and carry things with your upper body.

Examples of Move exercises include (in order of ascending difficulty):

Leg press

Squat

Split squat

Walking lunge

Walking lunge with rotation

Note: If you have a history of joint or lower back pain or have other restrictions due to health concerns (surgeries, orthopedic issues, etc.), exercise caution when making any change to or increasing your strength training plan. To prevent injury or complications, stay within the higher rep range of 15 to 25 and use light resistance. Check with your physician if you have questions or concerns.

PROGRESSION FOR STRENGTH TRAINING
When to Make Changes

If you crave variety, you can change your workout each day or each week. Or you can stick with the same plan for several consecutive weeks, if you find something that you really like and feel is just the right challenge for you. We recommend making a change to your plan at least every 3 to 6 weeks to keep from becoming bored and to continually challenge your body with new exercises and different types of resistance.

What to Change

You can choose to change any of the variables we've outlined in this chapter. However, as you change one, it may affect others. To simplify the process, we have outlined some key relationships between variables (see below). We focus on difficulty and resistance because changes to these two variables drive changes in the others.

Changing the number of reps typically occurs as a *result* of changing difficulty or resistance, not the other way around, as you will see below.

Changing the number of sets performed is a matter of your time commitment and your fatigue. Don't continue a workout if you cannot maintain good form.

Changing frequency also depends on your time commitment and your personal preference.

If you increase difficulty:

Decrease resistance.*

Decrease reps at first and then increase reps as you become stronger and more skilled.

Increase rest period as needed to maintain good form. In most cases, 1 to 2 minutes will suffice.

Decrease speed of movement. Only increase the speed of the movement after you master the exercise and only if fast movement is appropriate for the exercise you are doing.

If you increase resistance:

Decrease the difficulty.*

Decrease reps at first, and then increase reps as you become stronger.

Increase rest period as needed to maintain good form. In most cases, 1 to 2 minutes will suffice.

Decrease speed of movement. Only increase the speed of the movement after you master the exercise and only if fast movement is appropriate for the exercise you are doing. Keep in mind that it is often impossible to move a heavy resistance quickly *and* safely.

*When you increase the difficulty of an exercise that uses external resistance such as a bench press (for example, by doing a bench press on a stability ball), you can decrease the resistance by using a lighter weight. However, if you increase the difficulty of a body-weight exercise (for example, by going from modified pushups on your knees to regular pushups or from squats to squats on a BOSU), you have no way to decrease the resistance. When you increase the difficulty of a body-weight exercise, decrease the reps and build back up as you get stronger.

CHAPTER 26

Rejuvenation

Rejuvenation refers to restoring and refreshing your mind, body, and spirit after a busy day or in the midst of life's stresses and challenges. It is an essential, though often overlooked, part of your exercise plan. It will help keep you feeling motivated; improve your exercise performance by speeding up your recovery from workouts and making sure you are able to move through a full range of motion; and reduce your chances of an injury or illness that would sideline your exercise program.

Some active ways to refresh and renew include:

Body scanning	Stretching
Breathing exercises	Tai chi
Pilates	Yoga

Some more passive methods of rejuvenation include:

Baths (warm baths for relaxation and ice baths for recovery from workouts)	Hot tubs
	Meditation
	Saunas
Cold packs	Sleep
Heat packs	

BENEFITS OF REJUVENATION

When you face a challenge, whether it is moving to a new house or apartment, changing jobs, handling relationship problems, or changing ingrained eating and exercise behaviors, you might experience one of three different reactions. Here are examples of each type of reaction as it relates to changing to a healthy lifestyle and losing weight.

Agitation and dismissal. You feel inadequately equipped to deal with the issue at hand, resentful that you have to make changes, or frustrated and embarrassed that others "get it" and you don't, all of which make you withdraw from the challenge rather than take it on. When it comes to weight loss, you don't feel like it's worth it to put any real effort into the task. You are likely to quit your plan when it doesn't seem to be working for you.

Holding tight and pushing through. Your motivation is high and you charge full steam ahead, bound and determined to overcome the challenge. When it comes to exercise, you ignore fatigue as well as aches and pains because you're bent on sacrificing to reach your goals. You might feel angry with yourself for giving in to fatigue or push until you're sick or injured. Your weight-loss efforts are typically all-or-nothing affairs; you do everything to a T for as long as you can stand it, and then you stop when your momentum gets interrupted by burnout, injury, or simply not being able to do everything you think you "should."

Pausing and gaining perspective. You are aware of your emotions and the sensations of your body as you experience them, not just in hindsight. You do not think of going back to the basics as failing; you don't return to those basics because you are inadequate or deficient, but because there is something to be seen anew with each return and this increases your skill while making the process richer. You understand that an illness or injury is not your body fighting against you, but rather your body telling you that it needs to heal. You understand that adapting to new challenges is a major key to sticking to your exercise plan and to weight-loss success. And you know that adapting requires listening to and embracing your body, as well as understanding your strengths and your limitations.

Attending to Rejuvenation increases the likelihood that pausing and gaining perspective will become your preferred reactions. Doing so increases your chances of being an active person for the rest of your life because you'll give yourself the time to learn new tasks, to try and try again, and to embrace the journey of being active rather than only focusing on the goal of losing weight.

Here are several other key ways that Rejuvenation helps you stay active and healthy.

Decreased risk of injury

Improved recovery from workouts

Improved range of motion

Increased immune system function

Sharpened mental acuity and focus

Increased capacity for relaxation

Increased sense of enjoyment

HOW TO: REJUVENATION

The Rejuvenation activities listed on page 212 can be performed daily or even multiple times within the same day. They can be as quick as a 1- to 5-minute meditation between meetings or as long as a 60-minute yoga class or Pilates session.

CYT COMPONENTS OF REJUVENATION

The components of Rejuvenation refer to the restorative effect that you are seeking.

Lengthen: If you are like most people in the modern world, you sit for large parts of the day slumped over a desk and craning your neck to see a computer screen. This can lead to overstretching your back muscles and shortening the muscles in the front of your shoulders and chest, which can lead to back, shoulder, and neck pain, as well as headaches. Exercise can also lead to short, tight muscles if you do not regularly lengthen them. Lengthening activities—including stretching, yoga, Pilates, and massage— help maintain a healthy range of motion in the joints of your feet, ankles, knees, hips, spine, arms, hands, shoulders, and neck.

Position: This refers to your posture, which is improved by working your core muscles as you do in activities like yoga, deep breathing techniques, Feldenkrais Method, Pilates, and tai chi. It also refers to the way you carry yourself as you walk and the way you sit at your desk.

The mind and body are inextricably and beautifully connected; affect one, and you affect the other. Your attitude also affects your posture. You have probably noticed how you sink into your chair if you feel embarrassed and how you "swell" with pride at a job well done. Likewise, your position affects your attitude. Sitting and standing taller may just give you a little boost in confidence.

Meditate: This refers to your ability to sit still and stay present in your body. Focusing on your breath or heartbeat and engaging in other mind-quieting techniques have been proven to help reduce stress and heighten sensitivity to physical and emotional signals. Tuning in to important cues like hunger, satiety, pain, and exertion can help keep you from overeating or overexercising. And mindfulness can help you better cope with emotions and stress that may be driving you to overeat. Techniques for turning your attention inward include meditation, some forms of yoga, a mindful body scan (see "Tune In to Your Body" on page 98), and the silent recitation of a powerful, positive phrase or mantra.

Renew: You achieve this through "passive" therapies that recharge your body and mind. Enjoy a massage to relax tired muscles and help them recover from the stress of your day or the demands of a tough workout. Use restful heat by applying a hot pack or soaking in a hot tub or sauna to help your muscles and your mind relax. Cold therapies, such as a simple ice pack, can also reduce the inflammation of joints and muscles. Finally, nothing replaces regular, deep, and restful sleep. It is directly connected to lower levels of stress, better recovery from workouts, and lower body weight.

Note: Follow the appropriate guidelines for using hot tubs and saunas and use them for rejuvenation only. They are not aids to weight loss; do not attempt to "sweat off" weight.

PROGRESSION FOR REJUVENATION

Rejuvenation is meant to provide recovery from the stresses in your life, both physical and emotional. As such, the effort required may range from soothing and comfortable (such as a gentle stretch, Swedish massage, or deep breathing) to demanding (such as holding a yoga pose, actively stretching with props like resistance bands or foam rollers, or a deep tissue massage). Matching the experience to your level of fitness, skill, and physical tolerance is essential to getting what you want and need from your Rejuvenation. But you also need to match the experience to your *intention.*

Intention refers to the state of mind with which you enter the experience and your attitude toward what is being offered. Do you go into the session or class with the hope of getting a tough workout, or are you seeking something that is restorative? Even the most soothing yoga class will only produce agitation if it is not something you enjoy and embrace. And if it is a hard effort you're looking for, you can find it in yoga, Pilates (particularly with the reformer machine), and many of the "fusion" classes (like those that combine yoga and cardio) that are now available. But keep in mind that when you aim for a *workout*, it may not fall under the heading of Rejuvenation.

Aim to do some Rejuvenation every day. The more time-consuming options, like yoga classes, are limited by your time and motivation. Little things, like light stretching or quiet time to reflect and meditate, can make a big difference and are easy to incorporate into even the busiest day. Enjoy!

PUTTING IT ALL TOGETHER

We hope you will look at the Healthy Exercise Guidelines as a blueprint to becoming an active person.

You now know that being active literally means being willing and able to move. You know that cardio doesn't have to be complicated: It all starts with finding an amount and a pace that feel good to you, and if you want more of a challenge, then you go a little longer or a little harder. And the strength training options are not as scary as you thought; they can actually be inviting, as long as you know how to break them down into a few easy components.

Finally, as we have mentioned before, it doesn't matter how much you exercise now if you don't stick with it later. Ironically, to stay consistent with exercise you need to learn to take time off from it to relax and rejuvenate. Rejuvenation is just as important as any cardio and strength training exercise you perform.

We encourage you to use everything you've learned here about fitness in whatever way works for you, and don't be afraid to change it up as your life, abilities, and needs evolve. And most of all, enjoy being an active person!

PART 6

DISCOVERING YOUR POSITIVE INNER COACH

Now it's time to create your own wellness vision and set goals of your own! We hope the guidance that we provide in this section is meaningful to and supportive of you on your journey toward lasting weight loss and lifestyle change.

Some of you may have established some goals already, and that is fine. We hope that if you have "test driven" some of them, you have learned a lot about what works and what does not work for you.

The trial-and-error nature of setting and attaining goals will continue even after you are skilled at and comfortable with the process. Learning about yourself and what works for you and making adjustments in your thinking is more than just a smart way to go about changing your behaviors—it is a fundamental part of your long-term success.

"Discovering Your Positive Inner Coach" is divided into two sections. "Section 1: The Coach's Mental Toolbox" contains coaching tools and strategies intended to help you attain each of the powerful new ways of thinking outlined in "Part 3: The Five Stepping-Stones to Change" (see page 44).

In "Section 2: Vision Building and Goal Setting," you will learn the essential skills you need to set and adjust your goals as your circumstances change, your tastes in food transform, your physical fitness improves, and your relationship with eating and exercise evolves.

We have chosen this order because we believe that attaining the ways of thinking outlined in "The Five Stepping-Stones to Change" is vital if you are to stick to the goals you set. However, don't feel obligated to finish your journey through the Stepping-Stones before you set any goals.

If you set goals and don't reach them, revisit and adjust them so that they are more realistic and keep you moving forward. Changing your thinking is a process; the more closely your thinking aligns with the five Stepping-Stones, the greater your chances of maintaining your healthy behaviors and reaching your goals.

It's time to make some changes! Dive into Part 6 and enjoy this exciting part of your journey. As always, if you would like to pursue help outside of what *Coach Yourself Thin* can provide, check out the Resources on page 273 for suggestions. It's never necessary to go it alone.

CHAPTER 27

Tools for Expecting Greatness

This Stepping-Stone is equal parts realistic planning and expansive vision-building. The following tools will help you prepare yourself for lasting change and build a powerful vision for success.

PERSONAL STRENGTHS

Expecting to succeed is an important step toward actually succeeding. A big part of expecting success with lifestyle change is believing that you are capable of achieving the change that you want for yourself. You also need to be fully invested in and committed to the pathway you choose to follow. Use the statement and ranking system below to assess your current level of belief about your future success with healthy lifestyle change. Fill in the blanks with any change you envision making in your life, like:

"I believe I can make healthy food choices most of the time."

"I believe I can exercise consistently."

"I believe I can lose weight in a healthy way and keep it off."

Or, come back to this exercise once you have established your 3-month goals and/or weekly goals (see page 253) and apply this exercise to those goals.

Apply the following statement to each change or specific goal that you want to assess:

I believe I can [*insert change or specific goal*].

1. Strongly disagree

2. Disagree

3. Neither disagree nor agree

4. Agree

5. Strongly agree

If you answer at a level of 3 or below, consider using the exercise below to help you increase your confidence so that you can make the change or reach the specific goal in question.

The level of belief you have about achieving a particular change is an expression of your confidence in your ability to bring about that change. You can utilize your personal strengths to help increase your confidence. List five of your personal strengths below. Ask for suggestions from people you trust to be truthful (see "Discover Your Inner Circle" on page 73) and/or refer to the personal strengths tool in Resources (page 273) if you have doubts about your strengths or cannot think of five.

My personal strengths:

_____

_____

_____

_____

_____

Which strengths are relevant to helping you make the change you listed above?

What are some situations in which you have used these strengths in the past?

How could you use these strengths to help you achieve the change in question?

Go back and revisit the statement above. How did listing your personal strengths affect your belief/confidence that you can bring about this change in your life? If you are still at a 3 or below on the scale, consider amending your intended change to increase your belief/confidence that you can attain it. (See "Writing Powerful, Personal and Effective Goals" on page 250 for help writing more achievable goals.)

DECISIONAL BALANCE

It is entirely possible to be confident that you can make a change, yet not be ready to take on the effort required.

According to the groundbreaking work of James Prochaska and colleagues,[1] your readiness to change occurs in six defined stages: precontemplation, contemplation, preparation, action, maintenance, and termination.

You can assess your readiness to change by responding to the four statements below. Keep in mind that "the problem" mentioned in the questions may refer to an area of your life you want to change or a SMART goal you have set.

Respond either yes or no to the following statements:

1. I solved my problem more than 6 months ago.
2. I have taken action within the past 6 months to solve my problem.
3. I am intending to take action in the next month.
4. I am intending to take action within the next 6 months.

No to all statements = precontemplation

No to 1 to 3 and yes to 4 = contemplation

No to 1 and 2, yes to 3 and 4 = preparation

No to 1, yes to 2 = action

Yes to 1 = maintenance

If you are ready to begin your journey, then you have progressed through precontemplation and contemplation and have arrived in at least the preparation phase (intending to change within the next month). Perhaps that is why you picked up *Coach Yourself Thin*. You're hoping to use the information you find here to you bridge the gap from preparation into action. Or maybe you are in the action stage (change has begun within the past 6 months) and you are looking for help sticking with your plan (maintenance).

If you are not ready to make a healthy changes (precontemplation or contemplation), we believe that *Coach Yourself Thin* can be an important part of your progress to preparation and then into action; hearing stories about people who have been successful and witnessing the impact of healthy changes on people's lives can help you move forward. However, to move forward it is also essential that the change hold some value and importance for you. The exercise below can help you evaluate the personal value and importance of making a particular change.

Often you will feel ambivalent about making a change in your life. You can examine this ambivalence by looking at how the change will impact you in both positive and negative ways. This will help you evaluate objectively whether the change you're considering is right for you.

Consider the pros and cons of making the change you identified above. Compare them to the pros and cons of continuing on your current path. To help you make this comparison draw four boxes on a piece of paper, one each for:

Pros of making the change: What is exciting about it, what will it make better in your life, what are you looking forward to?

Cons of making the change: What will you have to sacrifice, what will you miss, what upsets you about making the change?

Pros of not making the change: What do you like about your current way of living with regard to this area of your life, what will you be happy you don't have to give up?

Cons of not making the change: What will you miss out on by continuing on your current path with regard to this area of your life?

Fill these boxes with as much information as you can about the change you listed above, and then review your responses.

What did you discover about your feelings regarding this change?

Go back and revisit the readiness assessment above. How did listing the pros and cons of your intended change affect your readiness? Did you find that the change is more valuable and important than you imagined and you are feeling more prepared to change? Or did you find that you are still in precontemplation or contemplation? If you are still not prepared to change, consider amending the change in question to make it more exciting and meaningful. (See the vision building exercise below as well as "Writing Powerful, Personal and Effective Goals" on page 250 to help with this process.)

CREATING A WELLNESS VISION

Your wellness vision is what you would see if you were to look into a crystal ball and see your ideal future self. Your vision does not have to be completed within a certain time frame. Consider what you are *aiming for,* and you can think about how to get there later. Make your picture as clear and thorough as you can. Be specific about what is important to you and what you want out of life; think about the person you want to be, the places you want to go, and the things you want to do. This is much more powerful than saying, "I want to be toned" or "I want to be healthy."

To find your true vision, answer these coaching questions to help identify your personal motivators.

What kind of person do I want to be? How do I want to see myself and how do I want others to see me? How would my ideal epitaph read?

How and where do I want to live? Where do I want to travel? How do I want to spend my days? What are the things I'd do if I had unlimited time and resources? What do I want to accomplish before I die?

What do I want to do more often or better? What is something I miss doing from when I was thinner, healthier, and more active?

Examples of Wellness Visions

Below is our client Pennie's first attempt to clarify her wellness vision.

With this journey of wellness that I have undertaken, I want to reach that realm of thinking that allows me to feel good about myself both physically and mentally. Being physically fit and healthy will allow me to enter the next chapter of my life with my family and experience the happiness that comes from being able to enjoy them. I will be the person I always wanted to be: active and engaged in life.

We encouraged Pennie to look a bit deeper by asking herself the following coaching questions:

What do I mean when I say, "feel good about myself both physically and mentally"?

What does it mean to me to be "physically fit"? What about "healthy"?

How will I be more "engaged in life"?

With these questions, Pennie came up with a more refined and powerful vision.

I am able to set ambitious running goals and achieve them, running faster than ever before. I'm a strong competitor within my age group. My strength sessions make me look and feel strong, give me an adrenaline rush, and complement my goal of success in my running.

I feel incredibly healthy and have none of the typical medical issues that are supposed to occur "at my age." I eat "clean," choosing mostly whole foods that give me more energy. I'm passionate about my food choices because they help fuel and heal my body.

I feel comfortable in my own skin. I'm proud of how far I've come and I like what I see when I look in the mirror. I feel good about where I am in my life because I'm able to accomplish so much more now, in all aspects of my life, than I could when I began my journey. I am the person I always wanted to be, active and engaged in doing the things I love.

Being physically fit and healthy allows me to enter the next chapter of my life with full confidence that I will be able to enjoy my family and reach our dreams.

Ask yourself probing questions to discover the heart of your wellness vision. Imagine describing your vision to a complete stranger and wanting to leave absolutely no doubt as to what it is that you want out of life.

CHAPTER 28

Tools for Regaining Your Balance

In today's world, it is very likely that your sense of balance has been skewed by the myths and misconceptions sold to you by the weight-loss industry. Regaining your balance requires that you find a way to make healthy choices while navigating a torrent of unhealthy ones. These tools will help you rediscover some healthy options you may not have considered before and help you find the time and energy to fit them into your life.

TAKING INVENTORY

A big step toward regaining your balance is to take inventory of all of the healthy foods that you enjoy or are willing to eat and to pinpoint activities that you can imagine yourself pursuing during the coming year. After choosing foods from the Healthy Food Preferences list below, create a master shopping list to keep in your wallet or on your phone; that way, you'll always have it handy when you go shopping. Using this list, establish daily and weekly goals for increasing your intake of healthy foods. Likewise, review the Activity Preferences list and build goals around the activities you are currently doing or would like to do.

Healthy Food Preferences

Fruits and Veggies

Fruits

Apples

Applesauce, no sugar added

Apricots

Bananas

Blackberries

Blueberries

Cantaloupe

Cherries

Dates

Figs, fresh

Fruit cocktail, in juice

Grapefruit

Grapes

Honeydew

Kiwifruit

Mangoes

Nectarines

Oranges

Papayas

Peaches, fresh or canned, in juice

Pears

Pineapple, fresh or canned, in juice

Plums

Prunes

Raisins

Raspberries

Strawberries

Tangerines

Watermelon

Raw Vegetables

Alfalfa/clover sprouts

Bean sprouts

Broccoli

Cabbage

Carrots

Cauliflower

Celery

Cucumbers

Green onions/scallions

Lettuce (iceberg, green or red leaf, romaine, or mixed salad greens)

Onions (red, white, yellow, or Vidalia)

Peas, sugar snap

Peppers (red, green, yellow, or orange bell)

Radishes

Spinach

Tomatoes, fresh

Cooked Vegetables

Asparagus

Beans (green, fresh, or steamed)

Beans (green or canned)

Beets

Broccoli

Brussels sprouts

Cabbage

Carrots

Cauliflower

Celery

Greens (collard, kale, mustard, turnip, or Swiss chard)

Mixed greens

Mushrooms

Spinach

Summer squash (yellow)

Tomato sauce

Turnips

Zucchini

Healthy Fats

Nuts (almonds, Brazil nuts, cashews, hazelnuts, peanuts, pecans, pistachios, or walnuts)

Nut butters (almond butter, peanut butter, or cashew butter)

Seeds (flaxseeds, pumpkin seeds, sesame seeds, or sunflower seeds)

Seed butters (sesame seed butter/tahini or sunflower seed butter)

Avocadoes

Olives

Olive oil

Canola oil

Virgin coconut oil

Salmon

Sardines

Tuna, albacore

Eggs labeled as source of omega-3s

Healthy Carbohydrates

Fruits and vegetables (see list above)

Winter squash (butternut, acorn, Hubbard, spaghetti, delicata, etc.)

Sweet potatoes

Beans (black, pinto, navy, great northern, lentils, kidney, split peas, etc.)

Peas, green, fresh or frozen

Edamame (green soybeans)

100 percent whole wheat bread (3 grams of fiber per 100 calories)

100 percent whole grain crackers, like Wasa or Ryvita

Brown rice

Quinoa

Oatmeal

Popcorn

High-fiber cereals (5+ grams of fiber per cup)

Low-fat dairy products (yogurt, low-fat or nonfat cottage cheese, skim milk, or kefir)

Healthy Protein

Chicken breast

Turkey breast

Salmon

Shrimp

Tuna, canned

Whitefish (tilapia, perch, flounder, cod, etc.)

Cottage cheese, nonfat

Eggs

Egg whites

Milk, skim

Soymilk, low-fat

Beans (black, pinto, navy, great northern, lentils, kidney, split peas, etc.)

Vegetarian burgers (whole foods–based)

Activities Preferences

Aerobic dance (all styles)

Aikido

Archery

Badminton

Baseball

Basketball

Bicycling

Bocce

Bowling

Boxing

Calisthenics

Camping

Canoeing

Capoeira

Climbing

Cricket

Croquet

Curling

Dancing

Diving

Enjoy a playground

Fencing

Fishing

Footbag

Football

Frisbee

Functional training, e.g., TRX, stability ball, BOSU

Golf

Gymnastics or tumbling

Handcycling

Hiking

Hopscotch

Horseback riding

Horseshoes

Hula hoop

Ice-skating

In-line skating

Jogging

Jujitsu

Judo

Jumping rope

Karate

Kayaking

Kickboxing

Kung fu

Mountain biking

Nia

Nordic walking

Paddleball

Pilates

Racquetball

Rafting

Rock climbing

Roller-skating

Rowing

Running

Sailing

Scuba diving

Situps

Sledding

Snorkeling

Skiing, downhill or cross-country

Snowshoeing

Soccer

Softball

Spinning

Squash

Stretching

Swimming

Tai chi

Tae Bo

Tae Kwon Do

Table tennis

Tennis

Trampoline

Volleyball

Walking

Water aerobics

Water-skiing

Weight lifting/strength training

Yoga

FINDING TIME

When you are structuring your schedule to accommodate your new lifestyle changes, it's important to make a distinction between *finding* time for yourself and *making* or *creating* time. You need to look at your schedule and *find* the time. We all have 24 hours every day to use as we see fit. What fills your day, therefore, are your priorities. If something is important enough to you, it gets done. Things that you'd like to get done, but that just aren't quite at the top of your priorities list, fall by the wayside.

At first glance, it may seem like you "have to" do many of the things in your life. But everything involves choice. You have chosen a path that includes the people with whom you surround yourself, your job, your location, and how you like to spend your time and resources. At any point, you could choose to give up any of these things and take a different path, and your values and beliefs help you decide which choices to make. No matter how trapped or "put upon" you feel, you have a choice. And a good way to ensure that you find time for taking care of *yourself* in spite of your busy schedule is to place a higher value on your health and fitness. If you value it, you will make it a priority and be more likely to find the time you have been looking for.

It's also important to acknowledge that circumstances affect you. None of us would choose to have our home swept away in a hurricane or be injured in an accident. And yet those things happen and influence what we prioritize, sometimes by changing what we feel we need in that moment or at that point in our lives; sometimes a shift in our circumstances will even change our core values and beliefs.

Below is an exercise to help you experience what it feels like to have your priorities shifted by your values.

How would you adapt if something happened in your life that required you to spend 45 minutes each day helping a good friend or significant other do something? Perhaps they need help dealing with issues at work or with health problems. It can be anything you can think of that would require time and effort from you.

Could you find the time and energy? Why?

If your answer to the above is no, then you're certainly too busy or tired to take on exercise or focus on healthy eating. In this case, an excellent next step is to take a look at your schedule and your surroundings and assess where you may be able to make changes that will allow you the time and energy to adopt a healthier lifestyle. (See "Creating Successful Environments" on page 69 and "Tools for Creating Successful Environments" on page 232.)

However, if you answered yes, it may very well be true that you would gladly put aside time for your loved one, but not for yourself.

In that case, it is important that you acknowledge that you're making a conscious choice not to make time for yourself and that you may not be ready, willing, or able to change at this point. An appropriate next step for you is to revisit "Tools for Expecting Greatness" on page 219.

DEFINING TREAT VERSUS CHEAT

We encourage you to establish ways to treat yourself, both with and without food, on a regular basis as part of your weight-loss program. The all-or-nothing mindset considers any deviation from the plan a "cheat," whereas the healthier 80/20 mindset thinks of a splurge as a "treat." This is a very important distinction: When you eat something you enjoy, you are not cheating anyone, nor are you doing anything wrong. Rather, a healthy splurge is a step toward making your weight-loss program more enjoyable and sustainable. You'll find that having guilt-free treats will help you feel more satisfied and remain consistent with your program.

When you look at a healthy treat by the numbers, you'll see that it has minimal impact over the course of a week. What may feel like a diet-busting 600-calorie splurge raises your average daily intake by less than 100 calories over the course of one week. These extra calories won't significantly slow your weight-loss progress if you are meeting your other weekly goals. You can break up your treat calories into several smaller treats or allow yourself one delicious dessert, a higher-calorie entrée, or a cocktail and a couple of bites of dessert.

Here are the guidelines for having treat calories.

1. Give yourself full permission to enjoy your treat without guilt.

2. Make the treat something you *really* enjoy; don't try to substitute something you *think* you should eat, instead.

3. Eat your treat as slowly as possible, allowing your taste buds to experience the full pleasure and awareness of what you are eating.

4. Practice feeling good that you are treating yourself *as part of* your program.

CHAPTER 29

Tools for Creating Successful Environments

Your immediate surroundings and the people in your life can be great allies in your journey, or they can make change nearly impossible. The following tools will help you take charge of your surroundings, ask for assistance and support when you need it, and be prepared for situations that could potentially knock you off track.

USING THE LAW OF DISPLACEMENT

To take charge of creating a successful environment to make healthy eating easier, begin by identifying a specific high-risk food or situation that you face with your eating program, either at home or at work. Then, think through each facet of what we call the Law of Displacement.

Omission: Avoid buying or having a specific trigger food nearby.

Line of Sight: Keep the trigger food out of view, tucked in a cupboard, drawer, or in another room.

Substitution: Choose a healthier food to replace the trigger food.

Use this formula to determine specific solutions that could work for you:

High-risk food or situation + Law of Displacement = Specific solution or strategy

Here are some examples of solutions you could come up with using the Law of Displacement.

At home: Late-night ice cream with your spouse or significant other.

- Late-night ice cream + Omission = Avoid buying the ice cream.
- Late-night ice cream + Line of Sight = Move to another room when your spouse or significant other eats ice cream.
- Late-night ice cream + Substitution = Eat a low-fat frozen yogurt or frozen fruit bar instead of ice cream.

At work: Pizza lunch on Friday.

- Pizza lunch + Omission = Choose to not order pizza, if the decision is within your control.
- Pizza lunch + Line of Sight = Avoid the break room where the pizza is served.
- Pizza lunch + Substitution = Pack a satisfying sandwich and yogurt, and eat this instead of pizza.

At work: Candy jar.

- Candy jar + Omission = Remove the candy jar altogether, if the decision is within your control.
- Candy jar + Line of Sight = Ask that the candy jar be kept in a cupboard instead of out in the open.
- Candy jar + Substitution = Bring something healthy to snack on whenever you get the urge to dip into the candy jar.

Your high-risk food or situation: _____

_____

+ Law of Displacement: _____

_____

= Specific solution or strategy: _____

WRITING AN ASSERTIVENESS LETTER

It can be very difficult to speak up for yourself. Our culture frowns on asking for help or putting yourself first. If you're female, you may have grown up seeing the women in your life as caregivers, and you may identify the caregiver role as one of your most important.

However, tactfully asking for what you need in order to live your life in a healthy way is essential. An Assertiveness Letter will go a long way toward communicating to the important people in your life exactly what it is that they can do to support you or to avoid putting obstacles in your way. Feel free to draft and edit this letter several times as you formulate precisely what you want to say and how you want to say it. You can deliver it to your loved ones in print form or use it as a script to rehearse what you'd like to say in person.

Your Assertiveness Letter may also just be a written catharsis for you—a way to get things off your chest without actually saying them aloud. If you're frustrated by a lack of support or outright sabotage (see page 73) from those around you, writing down your feelings can reduce your stress level and help keep the situation in perspective. This process may bring up even more anger or frustration, but keep in mind that writing it down is like counting to 10 when you're upset: It gives you time to think about it and to amend what you say before you say something you might regret.

Here are some guidelines for creating your Assertiveness Letter.[1]

- Brainstorm what you feel like you must have in order to be successful. Circle the things that stand out as most essential. (If they're all essential, then circle them all!)

- Who could help you arrange for these things to happen? What sort of help would you need? What would be an effective first step?

- Brainstorm some nonessentials that would make your journey easier, more fun, or more rewarding. These might include having your spouse exercise with you, signing up for a gym membership, planning family activities that involve movement, or purchasing some new kitchen appliances.

- Who could help you arrange for these things to happen? What sort of help would you need? If you had to choose one essential thing to happen first, which one would you choose?

- Brainstorm what you feel are sources of friction between you and the important people in your life.

- In what ways do your relationships and communication methods need to change to reduce this friction? What do you need to receive from others? What do you need to give in return?

Assertiveness Letter Example

Dear _____,

I have started eating healthier and exercising more consistently to improve my health and overall quality of life. It is clear to me that I will need support from you and all of my friends. What support means to me is having true care and concern for the well-being of another. Support takes many forms and looks different to different people. Some may thrive on praise, approval, and encouragement, whereas others don't want to have the extra attention or pressure.

It is difficult for family and friends to fully understand what support I need for my new lifestyle program. Many of the things that people do with good intentions are not supportive. Here are some examples of what is not helpful.

1. Lectures about weight loss and freely offered "constructive criticism" can feel demeaning, and unsolicited advice can be confusing. I *know* what to do to be successful, and it makes it more difficult to maintain my focus when others are offering unwanted and perhaps conflicting advice.

2. Despite your concern for me, my success does not depend on your "policing" my behavior. I, like most people, feel rebellious when I feel that others are watching and judging my every move. I am afraid that these behaviors will distract me from my program, making it more difficult for me to stick to my eating and exercise guidelines.

3. Please don't equate my eating and exercise program with deprivation. I will be tracking my food intake and making my own choices. I do not need to be on a deprivation diet in order to succeed. In fact, I have learned that eating too little can backfire and lead to overindulgence.

4. You can see that I've already made significant changes to my lifestyle, which have resulted in weight loss and increased

physical activity levels. Please don't be skeptical about the likelihood of my long-term success or my ability to recover from a setback. Your negativity may undermine my self-confidence.

5. Weight loss is a complicated process and may be slow and irregular. The scale is not the only measure of my progress, and I may prefer not to report the details of my weight loss because of the normal weight fluctuations and plateaus that I expect to experience. You may feel that your questions about my weight are supportive, but I may perceive them as pressure or criticism, and this may result in my feeling frustrated in not being able to report consistently better numbers every time you ask.

I know that you will try to do the best you can to help me, and I appreciate your efforts. I'd be happy to talk to you about ways that you can help encourage me. I know I can successfully follow my program with your help! Let's both work to keep the lines of communication open.

Yours in health, _____[1]

PREPARING FOR CHALLENGING SITUATIONS

Reflect now on challenging situations from your past that knocked you off your healthy eating and exercise track. Think about who was involved, where you were, and what emotions you were experiencing, as well as any specific foods or drinks that gave you trouble. Label the situation as either: (a) an anticipated situation, or one that you could have prepared for ahead of time, or (b) an unpredictable situation, or one that didn't allow much time, if any, to prepare. What could you have done differently in each situation?

Anticipated Situation

To navigate an anticipated situation, planning and problem solving are essential. Use the example that follows to help you brainstorm ideas that you can apply to similar situations in your own life.

It is announced that your work hours will be increasing significantly starting next month because your company has made cuts to staffing. What can you do to help keep yourself on track?

1. Write down an eating schedule based on set break times to follow as you transition to longer days.

2. Create a list of quick and healthy food ideas that you can shop for, and be prepared to make or pack so you have healthy choices at work.

3. Ask your boss about flex time so that you can get some exercise in the middle of the day, rather than waiting until after work, when you may be too tired.

4. Begin looking for other opportunities immediately if you believe that your health will likely suffer from working the extra hours.

Unpredictable Situation

Being creative and flexible can help you navigate challenging situations that you cannot anticipate. Use the example below to help you when you encounter unforeseen obstacles.

You get a phone call from a college friend who's passing through town and who invites you to dinner and drinks at a local pub tonight. Here are some of the tactics you might use to navigate this situation. Can you think of others?

1. You plan to have a snack 45 minutes before you meet up, to reduce your appetite and your chances of poor decision-making.

2. You go to the pub's Web site, find the menu, and decide in advance what you will order and how many drinks you will have.

3. You call your friend back and ask to change the dinner location to a healthier restaurant that offers more than burgers and fries.

4. You decide not to drink alcohol at the pub, knowing that drinking will likely throw you off track for the evening, as well as the next day or two. You are committed to drinking just water, focusing on making healthy food choices, and still having a great time!

CHAPTER 30

Tools for Being Unstoppable

A diet lasts until something comes along to knock you off track. A lifestyle lasts forever. The only "secret" to sticking to a healthy lifestyle is to become resistant to the obstacles and temptations that will inevitably show up in your path. The Tools for Being Unstoppable will create a more confident and resilient you that is less susceptible to setback but also more adept at getting up, dusting yourself off, and getting right back in action, when necessary.

MAKING SELF-TALK POSITIVE

By learning to "talk back" to your inner critic, you can take back your self-esteem and confidence. First, just listen to your self-talk. Is it positive? Encouraging? Do you demand a lot from yourself, but understand when you've given your best effort? Or is it negative and undermining?

Once you're aware of your self-talk, work on reframing one negative thought you have about yourself today. Write it down as soon as possible after it enters your mind and later, in a quiet moment, examine it.

How much truth is in what you said to yourself? If there is any truth, how would you frame that criticism if your good friend had the same flaws or was making the same mistakes as you?

If there is no truth at all, or if you have exaggerated a flaw or mistake, what is the truth?

Write down your reframed view of the flaw or mistake as if it were a rebuttal to your inner critic. For example, your reaction to seeing your reflection in the mirror might be, "Oh man, I can't believe how I've let myself go. I better get off my butt and do something about this." Then, upon reflection, you realize that you have actually made some changes to the way you eat, that your pants size has dropped, and that you are smiling more.

You say to your critic, "I'm looking better. I'm so happy that I've begun eating more vegetables and drinking more water during the day, because it shows!"

PREVENTING RELAPSE

You've worked hard to lose weight, and now it's time to take steps to protect your weight-loss progress and reduce the chances of a relapse with the green, yellow, and red flag system. With this system, you will establish specific daily and weekly goals at a time when you want to focus on weight maintenance. You can do this when you've reached your goal weight or anytime that you decide to take a break from weight loss, such as when you want to "try out" a particular weight to see how it feels and how successful you can be at maintaining it, or when you feel burned out with working on weight loss.

Establishing clear weekly goals will help you know when you're on track and when you're veering off course. It's much easier to catch yourself when you've slipped just a little than when you are way off course.

Green Flags

Even though you are not striving for the same goals as you were while losing weight, your new goals need to be just as defined. Write down your list of daily and weekly goals; these are your "green flags," and when you meet them, you are on a maintenance path.

Examples of Green Flags for Nutrition

You drink 48 or more ounces of water at least 5 days per week.

You eat two or three servings of fruit at least 5 days per week.

You eat three or more servings of vegetables at least 6 days per week.

You don't skip meals.

You eat healthy snacks.

You stay mindful of the food choices you make.

You choose small treats several times each week.

Examples of Green Flags for Exercise

You do 200 to 300 minutes of cardio per week.

You do two or three strength training sessions and three to five cardio sessions per week.

You burn 300 to 500 calories in each cardio session.

You keep your appointments for classes or training sessions.

You use a pedometer and reach 10,000 steps each day.

You stretch for 5 to 10 minutes after every workout.

You do exercise that makes you feel good and that you look forward to.

You listen to your body and stay injury-free.

Examples of Green Flags for Behavioral Awareness

You tune in to hunger and fullness signals.

You use the delay and nurture strategy (see page 247) when you feel the urge to eat.

You think about the pros and cons before making unhealthy food choices.

You use self-coaching to help yourself stay motivated.

You tune in to your emotions or thoughts.

You reframe negative self-talk with positive self-talk.

You consciously pursue enjoyable activities each day.

You use your support system regularly.

Yellow Flags

A relapse back to old habits is often very subtle. If you have a strong tendency to backslide, then define your "yellow" warning flags now so that you can catch yourself before you fall too far. Yellow flags are easier to correct if you catch them at the onset.

Yellow flags can be indicators that you are losing motivation or have made your health a lower priority. And in some cases, it could mean that you're trying too hard, which can lead to a mental or physical breakdown.

Examples of Yellow Flags for Nutrition

You are feeling tired of your food choices and notice that your meals lack variety.

Your cravings for sweets, salty foods, alcohol, and other treats increase.

You are doing less grocery shopping and food preparation.

You start missing a meal here and there and graze instead.

You are feeling more tempted by unhealthy foods at social engagements.

You are not meeting your goal for daily water intake.

You are drinking more alcohol than usual.

You are relying on caffeine to get you through the day.

You are eating fewer than two or three servings of fruits and vegetables per day.

Examples of Yellow Flags for Exercise

You feel unmotivated and have to drag yourself to the gym.

You are bored while working out and watch the clock constantly.

You are cutting your workouts short.

You let work get in the way of exercise more often.

You frequently miss a workout when it's not a planned rest day.

You're occasionally going more than 3 days between workouts.

You can't reach your typical speed or level.

You can't lift the same weights for the same number of reps as you could before.

You hit the snooze button and sleep through workouts.

Examples of Yellow Flags for Behavioral Awareness

You are not planning ahead to navigate difficult situations.

You are forgetting to use the delay and nurture strategy when you feel the urge to eat.

You are not thinking about the pros and cons very often before making unhealthy food choices.

You are not using self-coaching to help yourself stay motivated.

You are not paying much attention to your emotions or thoughts.

You are not noticing or reframing negative self-talk with positive self-talk.

Red Flags

Seeing red flags pop up on a regular basis means that you're quickly reverting back to your old lifestyle, if you're not already there.

Examples of Red Flags for Nutrition

You notice that you're not paying attention to your food, and you've stopped tracking it altogether.

You are bored with your diet and feel restricted by your food choices.

You are eating two or fewer servings of fruits and vegetables each day.

You are drinking fewer than 4 cups (48 ounces) of water on most days.

You are drinking more than one alcoholic drink on most days.

You are using junk food and caffeine as pick-me-ups.

You've stopped weighing yourself to avoid the truth.

You are skipping meals and snacks.

You are keeping a lot of trigger foods at home and in your line of vision.

Examples of Red Flags for Exercise

You miss an entire week of exercise.

You drop out of an exercise class or group.

You quit meeting with a personal trainer.

You don't renew your gym membership.

You have a nagging injury and are not doing anything proactive to make it better.

Examples of Red Flags for Behavioral Awareness

You are blaming yourself for your struggles and shortcomings.

You are not consciously pursuing enjoyable activities each day.

You are letting self-care go, including sleep habits, health, grooming, or other physical needs.

You are not relying on support from others.

Putting It All Together

The perfect time to create your green, yellow, and red flag system is when your motivation is high and you are determined to be successful with weight maintenance. Don't wait until you are struggling; rather, take the time to follow the steps below to create your flags and your action steps ahead of time.

Step 1: Make a list of your green, yellow, and red flags. Identify at least 2 flags from each of the three categories and each of the three colors—in other words, two green nutrition flags, two green exercise flags, and two green behavior awareness flags and the same for the other two colors.

Step 2: Review your yellow flags and identify corrective steps you can take when they pop up.

Step 3: Review your red flags and think about what steps you would take to get back with your program if you were to wake up and find yourself surrounded by red flags one day in the future.

You may be able to take the steps needed to get back on track on your own, or you may ask a trusted friend, counselor, personal trainer, or coach to help you. The steps you take don't need to be complicated; just make sure you have a plan in place.

Yellow flag: You are eating fewer than two servings of fruit per day.
   Action: Schedule time to go the market, buy enough fruit to last until your next scheduled market trip, and track your intake every day with the goal of getting your two servings in by the midafternoon.

Yellow flag: You are hitting the snooze button and sleeping through workouts.

Action: Plan a walk, run, or other physical activity with a friend so you *have* to get up.

Red flag: You are skipping meals and snacks.
   Action: Start tracking your meals for the week by joining a health and diet Web site.

Red flag: You miss an entire week of exercise.
   Action: Call your walking partner and arrange a date and time to get back on track.

BEING THANKFUL

Thinking about the things you are thankful for in your life has a powerful affect on your attitude. Gratitude can make you feel happier, give you purpose and help you through tough times. From a weight loss perspective, it can increase your resilience to obstacles to living a healthy life and help you stick to healthy behaviors even when you're facing temptations and stress.

The practice of writing down what you are thankful for will help you increase your awareness of and draw motivation from the positive things in your life. For one week, at the end of each day journal at least three things that:

* You believe went well for you
* You were successful in achieving
* You are happy about
* You are grateful for
* Show specific skills/strengths (like planning, for example) on your part

At the end of the week, look back over your list. How does the list of things you are thankful for affect your overall attitude? How might this exercise affect your ability to stick to healthy choices on those days when it is tough to do so?

CHAPTER 31

Tools for Awakening Your Intuition

To finally achieve independence from the failed dieting efforts of your past, you must rely on intuition: an "immediate understanding without the evident use of conscious rational processes." To maximize your "health intuition," use the following tools to tune in to your body and mind and bring to bear all the skills you have learned in the preceding Stepping-Stones.

UNDERSTANDING YOUR BODY LANGUAGE

One of the most frequently asked questions we hear from our clients is, "How do I know if I'm exercising hard enough?" As we discussed in Part 5, this is not an easy question to answer because "enough" is very dependent upon fitness level, physical ability, limitations, personal motivation, and goals. But we can help you answer this question for yourself by teaching you how to listen to your body more effectively.

When you exercise, you will feel sensations in your muscles that you may not be familiar with if you've been sedentary for a very long time. Exertion can result in fatigue or a feeling that your muscles are burning or aching. This can come on quickly, even after walking up a flight of stairs, and it usually goes away quickly if you slow down or stop.

You can refer to the RPE scale (see page 195) to review the appropriate levels of effort for cardiovascular exercise.

Unlike the achiness or discomfort that comes from effort, soreness usually peaks 24 to 48 hours after exercise and goes away slowly, often over several days. You may feel tight or stiff, and stretching the sore muscle generally feels good.

Pain, on the other hand, is a clear signal that something is wrong. It can come on suddenly or it may develop over several days or even weeks, starting out feeling like soreness but slowly getting worse, rather than going away. It may be accompanied by swelling or discoloration. Some types of pain, like tendonitis, might feel okay once you are warmed up but get worse once you cool down from exercise (tendonitis is notoriously worse when you first wake up). Other types, like a stress fracture, can get worse as your exercise session progresses. The painful area might hurt to the touch and will often occur near a joint because ligaments and tendons are frequently involved. Pain that seems to be inside the joint itself, especially when accompanied by joint swelling, is a very clear sign to back off.

If you have soreness or tightness, go ahead and exercise and stretch well afterward. If you have pain, skip your exercise session or stop if you have already begun exercising. Find a form of exercise that does not exacerbate your symptoms or, if that is not possible, stop exercising altogether. If pain symptoms persist for more than 2 weeks despite taking some time off from exercise, check with your doctor and/or physical therapist.

Body Scan

This exercise[1] will help you become more in tune with the sensations your body is sending you, which will head off potential injuries. The breath is used as a bridge between mind and body; it will allow you to check in with your internal indicators to help you learn to fully acknowledge and experience the sensations of physical movement during your exercise session.

Begin in a comfortable position, either lying down or sitting with your feet firmly on the floor and your back straight.

Close your eyes and begin to take deep breaths, inhaling and exhaling through your nose, allowing your breath to have the sound quality of a gentle wave. This is accomplished by keeping your jaw relaxed, your lips lightly touching, and your breath audible as a "sigh of contentment" at the back of your throat.

Place your hands gently on your belly, allowing your breath to expand and contract your lungs and diaphragm. Feel your breath rise and fall like a wave ebbing and flowing. Do this for several breaths.

Bring your awareness to your feet. Imagine a bright, warm light spreading through the soles of your feet. Watch this light as it moves up into your ankles and calves; allow it to pool here, radiating warmth, for a few breaths.

Consciously move the light, with the breath, into your knees and legs. Allow it to rest for a few breaths, growing in brightness as your legs get very heavy and relaxed.

After a few breaths, move the light into your abdomen, allowing it to expand in all directions with a full, radiant luminosity. From here, ease the light fully into your torso, filling your body as it lengthens upward toward your throat.

Hold the light in your throat for several breaths, allowing its brilliance to increase until finally it rises and flows into your head, spreading its warmth behind your eyes, enabling the muscles of your face to completely relax in its caress.

Your brow should be smooth, your jaw loose at its hinge, the tips of your ears relaxed as your skull and each hair on your head embraces the sweet glow.

Your entire body is now filled with warm, heavy light. Permit your awareness to rest in the slight pause between each inhalation and exhalation. If thoughts enter your mind, let them float by as clouds in the sky, as you gently bring your awareness back to the growing space between the breaths.

Rest here, captivated by the sound of your soft, subtle breath, in the splendor of your own full light.

After several moments, invite a deeper breath through your mouth and nose. Stretch as desired and, if you're lying down, gently roll to your side. Using your hands, push yourself up to a seated position and allow your eyes to gently open. If you performed this exercise while seated, invite the deeper breaths, stretch, and gently open your eyes.

RAISING AWARENESS OF EMOTIONAL EATING

The next time you feel a strong urge to eat and you're aware that your "hunger" is emotionally driven, use this delay and nurture exercise.

First, agree to delay your urge to eat for the next 10 minutes, after which time you will decide if you still want something to eat. Take a couple of deep breaths and drink a glass of water.

Body Language and Hunger Signals

In the same way that it is necessary to tune in to your body's signals as you move and exercise, it's also beneficial to tune in to your body's cues before, during, and after you eat. Take time to gauge your hunger. (See Hunger and Fullness Scale on page 135.) Doing this regularly will help heighten your awareness of your body's signals throughout the day and enable you to adjust your food intake more intuitively.

Next, think about how you can nurture yourself in the coming 10 minutes. Consider taking a shower; moving into another, more relaxing room; turning off the television if it is on; putting on your favorite music; playing a musical instrument; doing something that occupies your hands and requires focus, such as quilting, drawing, painting, writing a letter to a friend, or journaling; crawling into bed with a good book; or lighting a few candles and taking a time out for yourself.

If, after 10 minutes, you still desire something to eat, go ahead and have something. Check in with yourself to see if you would be satisfied with a healthier version of what you had in mind.

By performing this exercise, you have successfully raised your awareness about emotional eating, even if you end up choosing to have a snack. Take a few minutes to journal what you felt during this exercise.

Creating a Healthy Vortex

Write down at least 10 victories, other than losing weight, that you would like to experience in the coming year as a direct result of eating healthier, exercising more consistently, and making other positive changes. Here is a list of possible ideas.

My Victories Are That I . . .

- Have more energy
- Am sleeping better

- Experience less physical pain
- Am more physically fit
- Have reduced my intake of medications
- Have more confidence
- Go out more often with friends
- Have started dating
- Find healthy foods appetizing and enjoyable
- Have learned to cook some great, satisfying new meals
- Have found a tremendous support group
- Have stood up for myself, asking for what I need in order to live a healthy life

The next step of the exercise is to create your own Healthy Lifestyle Vortex in a short paragraph, connecting all of your victories in a creative story that you could be telling this time next year. Think about the concept of the vortex as a whirlwind: In terms of lifestyle, a healthy vortex is a way of life regarded as irresistibly engulfing because one healthy behavior or victory leads to more and more positive changes in your life.

Here's an example using many of the victories from the list above.

I used to drag myself out of bed every morning, but after I made some key changes to my eating and started drinking more water, my *energy* skyrocketed and I noticed that my *headaches disappeared*. Maybe this inspired me to start *exercising regularly*, or maybe it was that I was *sleeping better*. My *attitude improved* and I started feeling *more confident* about myself. My *friends noticed* the changes, and I started saying yes to going out more often with friends and *on dates*. Feeling better each day and being able to climb stairs without getting out of breath (being *more physically fit*) is incredible in itself, but I've also been able to *get off of two medications* in less than a year!

Parts of your story may resonate enough that you feel they could add inspiration and power to your wellness vision (see page 223). If so, rewrite your wellness vision to include the victories that you now foresee thanks to creating your own Healthy Lifestyle Vortex.

CHAPTER 32

Writing Powerful, Personal, and Effective Goals

Everyone likes to think about exciting outcomes. If you envision yourself as physically fit and capable, you may be working toward walking up all five flights of stairs to your apartment. If you see yourself as an athlete, perhaps you're training for a 10-K. Or maybe your vision is sharing romantic and exciting vacations with your significant other, and the outcome you want most is walking through a museum without worrying about your knees giving out. But you may not have given much thought to the behaviors that will help you arrive at those outcomes.

Your behaviors are made up of the little daily choices you make: your decision to exercise for 20 minutes, eat a healthy breakfast, or drink water instead of soda. And unlike the eventual outcomes (such as body weight or your 10-K time), you have immediate and powerful control over almost all of your health-related behaviors.

Unfortunately, the outcomes you originally had in mind may not directly follow your behaviors. For example, you can manage your exercise and eating plan just like you imagined and still not lose the number of pounds that you believe you should. This may be difficult for you to accept, but realistically you only have two choices. We call them the "diverging pathways," and you can only choose one.

1. You can hit your behavioral goals and lose the weight that your body is capable of losing, keeping in mind that this may not match your original weight-loss goal. You end up with the best outcome you can

achieve given your genetics, responsibilities, obligations, skills, limitations, and determination.

2. You can stick with your old behaviors or bounce from diet plan to diet plan, and you'll be whatever weight the diet roller coaster leads you to.

On one level, settling for your body's capabilities is hard to swallow. But at the same time, it can be incredibly empowering. If you set healthy, balanced goals and control the things you can, you'll never need to wonder whether you're doing enough or doing the right thing.

Your daily behaviors are like drops of water collecting in a bucket: You have to start with just one drop and then drop more in gradually, one by one. The trick is, the drops have to be steady enough so that one drop doesn't dry up before the next few arrive. And over time, they add up. Before too long, your bucket is overflowing with water.

SMART GOALS

To be effective, your goals have to be clear enough for you to follow, measurable enough for you to know when you've achieved them, and exciting enough that you are inspired to take on the challenge of pursuing them.

What Is SMART?

The SMART goal acronym (explained below) will help you create personal and powerful goals. Use "I will" statements to indicate your confidence that you will attain your goals.

SPECIFIC: The goals "I will exercise more" or "I will eat better this week" aren't specific. To be specific, you need to answer questions that probe into what you mean by these very general words, like, "What is more?" or "Better than what?" For example, "I will walk 30 minutes on Monday, Wednesday, and Friday this week" and "I will eat four servings of vegetables on 4 days this week" are very specific goals.

MEASURABLE: Measurable means that you can measure what you've done and keep track of your progress. "I will exercise hard 3 days per week" is not completely measurable because you have not defined "hard." The more specific a goal is, the more measurable it is. "On 3 days per week I will exercise on the treadmill for 30 minutes at a speed of 4.0 mph" is very measurable.

ACHIEVABLE: Keep your goals within reach. Setting impossible goals or goals that require too much sacrifice or effort to achieve will paralyze you. For example, "I will lose 5 pounds per week" is an unattainable goal for most people. And extreme goals like, "I will cut all refined sugar out of my diet" or "I will exercise 7 days per week" also set the bar too high.

To keep your goals achievable, stay focused on behaviors that are challenging to you but that you are confident you can reach. Ideally, you will feel confidence at a level of 4 or higher (on a scale where 1 is strongly disagree in your ability to achieve your goal and 5 is strongly agree). If you are at level 3 or below, consider rewriting your goal to make it more achievable and/or see "Tools for Expecting Greatness" on page 219.

REWARDING: Will it feel good to accomplish your goal? While goals that are too hard to achieve will likely frighten or frustrate you, a goal that is too easy will fail to inspire you. For example, "I will walk 5 to 10 minutes on 4 days per week" could prove uninspiring if you are fit enough to do much more. You may find yourself saying, "Why even bother?" Set goals that you feel great about reaching.

TIME-DEFINED: Establish goals that are both short-term and long-term and that are measured by specific time frames. We recommend both weekly and 3-month goals. For example, "I will eat at least five servings of fruits and vegetables on 2 or 3 days this week" is an excellent weekly goal that will help you build up to the 3-month goal, "I will eat at least five servings of fruits and vegetables 5 to 7 days each week."

Also keep in mind that goals with ranges can work better than dealing in absolutes. For instance, instead of, "I will go for a walk 5 days per week," create some flexibility in your goal: "I will go for a walk 3 to 5 days per week." Giving yourself some leeway will increase your chances of success.

How to Write a SMART Goal

Use open-ended coaching questions similar to the ones below to make your goals SMART.

Start out with a first draft of your goal:
I will exercise more consistently.

Coaching question: What form of exercise do I see myself doing?
I will do cardio more consistently.

Coaching question: What specific type of cardio will I do?
I will walk or ride my stationary bicycle more consistently.

Coaching question: How long will I aim to exercise each day?
I will walk or ride my stationary bicycle for 75 minutes per day consistently.

Coaching question: How realistic is it to aim for 75 minutes per day? How confident do I feel that I can do this consistently?
(If your confidence that you could exercise for this long is 3 or lower on a scale of 1 to 5, revise your goal to something more realistic.)
I will walk or ride my stationary bicycle for 30 minutes per day consistently.
(If your confidence is at a level of 4 or above and you feel challenged by this goal, then keep it as it is. If you do not feel challenged, you could actually increase the goal.)

Coaching question: How do I define "consistently"?
I will walk or ride my stationary bicycle for 30 minutes per day, 4 or 5 days a week.

Types of Goals

3-Month Goals

Your 3-month goals are the long-term goals designed to lead you slowly but surely to your vision. They are set far enough in the future to allow time for a meaningful change, yet not so far that you find them overly daunting or lose interest before you can reach them.

You want to be very confident that you can achieve any goal that you set, but that doesn't mean that you should play it totally safe. Because these goals do allow time for significant changes to take place, you should step outside your comfort zone a bit here and challenge yourself.

Weekly Goals

Just as 3-month goals are steps toward your wellness vision, your weekly goals are steps toward your 3-month goals. Because of the short time frame, these goals are much smaller in scope than your 3-month goals. To set realistic weekly goals, consider the small steps can you commit to changing immediately. Don't overlook the details by focusing on the larger picture too soon.

For example, you may want to begin counting calories but not have a good resource for how to do it accurately. In this case, a good first goal is to locate an online calorie counter or guidebook. Or you might want to go out and ride your old mountain bike, but then you roll it out of the garage and discover that the tires have deteriorated from sitting around and the chain is too rusty to work properly. In this case, a trip to the bike shop for maintenance and repair is a better first goal than aiming for a certain number of miles. And it certainly wouldn't do much good to plan 3 days at the gym if you are frightened and embarrassed that you don't know your way around the machines and weights. A session with a personal trainer would help you get started, so setting that up would be an excellent goal.

These details may seem trivial. However, it is precisely these sorts of logistical roadblocks that could keep you from taking the first steps toward change.

For more precision in your goals, use the same types of probing questions that we demonstrated in "How to Write a SMART Goal" on page 252. But in the case of weekly goals, it can be helpful to be specific down to the exact day or days of the week that you will complete a given goal. This works well when it is clear that pursuing your goal on a certain day or days will be more conducive to your success (days when you get to leave work earlier, you have a babysitter, or your spouse has activities of his or her own already planned), or when something you're aiming to do only occurs on particular days (such as exercise classes or support group meetings).

Allow yourself more flexibility if you feel "pinned down" or unnecessarily restricted by aiming for certain days.

CHAPTER 33

Bridging the Gap from Vision to Goals

Now that you have written a vision that you find exciting and empowering (refer to "Tools for Expecting Greatness" on page 219), learned the definition and importance of SMART Goals, and understood the function of 3-month and weekly goals, it's time to set your first 3-month goals.

STEP 1: PICK OUT THE "ELEMENTS" OF YOUR VISION

Look at your completed wellness vision (from the exercise on page 223) and define the distinct areas of your life that you believe are covered by your vision. This breaks your vision down into its elemental parts so that you can see clearly what it is you're aiming for.

Below is Pennie's full vision from page 224. In parentheses, we have noted sections that help illustrate areas that she might want to focus on. Keep in mind that a vision is personal and open to interpretation.

I am able to set ambitious running goals and achieve them. I'm a strong competitor in my age group. My strength training sessions make me look and feel strong and give me an adrenaline rush. **(Fitness)**

I feel incredibly healthy and have none of the typical medical issues that are supposed to occur at my age. **(Overall health)**

I eat "clean," choosing mostly whole foods that give me more energy. I'm passionate about my food choices because they help fuel and heal my body. **(Nutrition)**

I feel comfortable in my own skin. I'm proud of how far I've come and I like what I see when I look in the mirror. I feel good about where I am in my life because I'm able to accomplish so much more now than I could when I began my journey. I am the person I always wanted to be, active and engaged in doing the things I love in life. **(Self-esteem)**

Being physically fit and healthy allows me to enter the next chapter of my life with full confidence that I will be able to cherish my family and friends and truly enjoy the time we spend together. **(Relationships)**

STEP 2: DECIDE WHAT YOU WANT TO WORK ON

Now that you've broken down your vision into the various areas that are important in your life, you will need to select one to three on which to focus first. To help you do so, ask yourself the coaching questions below.

Which areas of my vision excite me the most?

Which areas of my vision do I most want to see become a reality?

Once you have decided which areas you want to focus your attention on first, take some time to consider which specific behaviors you want to change in each area.

STEP 3: SET 3-MONTH GOALS

Now that you've decided which areas you'd like to work on, set one to three 3-month goals in each area using the SMART goal guidelines (see page 252).

Note: We have recommended that you choose one to three areas of your vision to work on and that you set one to three 3-month goals for each area. However, if you were to choose the maximum number of each (three areas with three goals for each), you would end up with nine 3-month goals, a number we believe to be far too cumbersome to be effective for most people. Ideally, aim for the "sweet spot" of three to five *total* 3-month goals by prioritizing which behaviors you want to change first.

The following coaching questions are to be applied to each area you chose in Step 2 and will help you think about where you are now and where you want to be in 3 months.

What is my current status in this area of my life?

What behaviors can I challenge myself to change in this area of my life?

Here are a few possible 3-month goals based on the vision we shared above.

Related to the area of fitness

I will consistently run an average of 20 to 25 miles per week at a comfortable pace of 12 minutes per mile.

I will try one new strength training technique or style during the final week of each month and, if I like it, I will incorporate it into my regular strength routine the following month.

Related to the area of relationships

I will plan and lead two active family activities per month.

STEP 4: SET WEEKLY GOALS

Now that you have 3-month goals in place, it's time to begin working toward them. Again, using the Smart Goal guidelines on page 252, come up with a total of three to five exciting weekly goals for each 3-month goal. Keep in mind that this is just your first week's goals and, therefore, just your first steps toward your 3-month goals. You do not need to start working on all of your 3-month goals at the same time, and you will be able to make weekly changes as you progress, as outlined in Step 5 on page 258.

It's a good idea to revisit your wellness vision periodically; once or twice every 3 months is about right. Your perspective on your abilities, your strengths and weaknesses, and what direction you want to take in your life will evolve over time, and your goals should evolve, too.

Here are some examples of possible weekly goals.

3-Month Goal: "I will consistently run an average of 20 to 25 miles per week at a comfortable pace of 12 minutes per mile."

Weekly Goal: "I will run 2 miles on Tuesday and Thursday and 4 miles on Sunday this week, all at an average pace of 12 minutes per mile."

3-Month Goal: "I will try one new strength training technique or style during the final week of each month and, if I like it, I will incorporate it into my regular strength routine the following month."

Weekly Goal: "On Saturday, I will research new strength training techniques on the Web site my trainer recommended."

3-Month Goal: "I will plan and lead two active family activities per month."

Weekly Goal: "I will ask each member of my family to provide one idea for an activity that he or she would like to do as a group."

STEP 5: CONTINUALLY MODIFY YOUR GOALS

Your goals need to change as you change. One of the biggest drawbacks of most diet and exercise plans is that they give you the "how to" and then it never gets updated. What if you become a better cook and want to try out some new recipes? What if your fitness level eventually exceeds the workout you were aiming for? Using SMART goals instead of a "set in stone" plan allows you to make changes as you go.

In an ideal world, you would steadily increase your weekly goals each and every week until you hit your 3-month target. Plan to assess your progress at the end of every week and set your goals for the following week. Make sure your goals are measurable and specific and that they help you move one step closer to meeting your 3-month goal.

That having been said, "life happens" to all of us, and chances are that you will need to make changes to your weekly goals for a variety of reasons.

Below we discuss the four types of changes that you can use to modify your weekly goals based on what is going on in your life at any given moment. They provide the guidance you need to "up the ante" when things are going well, hold your own when you just need to stay on course, and lower the bar or even throw in the towel when a particular goal just isn't working.

And remember: As we mentioned above, weekly goals are not the only goals that might need an occasional tweak. You may also find it necessary to use the following modifications on a 3-month goal. You can make changes to a 3-month goal at any time, not just at the end of the 3 months! If you're progressing more slowly or quickly than you expected, or if a goal loses its appeal, make the necessary changes.

POSSIBLE NEXT STEPS

Maintain a Goal: You can maintain a goal that is working for you and that you find challenging but achievable.

Refine a Goal: You can change an existing goal. You might make a goal more challenging (raise the bar) if things are going really well or you have completed one step in the progression of a goal and are ready to take it to the next level. Or make a goal less challenging (lower the hurdle) if you are struggling to hit your target.

Add a New Goal: You can add a brand new goal when you are ready for a completely new challenge. Or you might add a goal when you need a different approach or strategy to help you achieve one of your weekly goals. Or perhaps a current goal is proving too difficult or is not motivating and you need to eliminate one of your weekly goals (see below) and add a goal that takes you in a different direction.

Eliminate a Goal: In some cases, you may choose to drop a goal completely. This may occur when you have set a goal in an area that you no longer find interesting or motivating or when you have achieved a goal and are ready to move on.

In Chapter 34, we demonstrate how to implement these modifications.

Case Study

This case study will take you back through all of the steps we outlined in Chapter 33. We've included the client's rationale for setting or modifying each goal, as well as the specific modification that was used.

Wellness Vision

I am strong and capable in my body as I age, and I am vital and energized all day long.

I am disciplined, and I respect the meaningful boundaries that allow a balanced life to flourish. I read for pleasure and participate in recreational activities with my family. I eat a clean, vegetarian diet, and I sleep well. Exercise is a consistent, seamless part of my life. I embrace these activities fully, as they support my physical, mental, and emotional self.

I am open to change and willingly refine my goals and the strategies that help me achieve them as new challenges come up. My job satisfaction remains incredibly high and my overall health is excellent.

As I move into the next phase of my life, I am an eager participant, gaining energy from my balanced approach to work, exercise, and time with my family.

STEP 1: PICK OUT THE "ELEMENTS" OF YOUR VISION

- I am disciplined, and I respect the meaningful boundaries that allow a balanced life to flourish. I gain energy from my balanced approach to work, exercise, and time with family. (**Life balance**)

- I am open to change and willingly refine my goals and strategies to help me achieve them as new challenges come up. (**Openness to change**)

- My job satisfaction remains incredibly high and my overall health is excellent. (**Overall health**)

- I am strong and capable in my body as I age, and I am vital and energized all day long. Exercise is a consistent, seamless part of my life. (**Fitness**)

- I eat a clean, vegetarian diet, and I sleep well. I read for pleasure and participate in recreational activities with my family. (**Behaviors that support my health**)

STEP 2: DECIDE WHAT YOU WANT TO WORK ON

Which elements of your vision excite you the most? Which elements of your vision do you most wish to see come true?

Fitness

- I am strong and capable in my body as I age, and I am vital and energized all day long.
- Exercise is a consistent, seamless part of my life.

Life Balance

- I am disciplined, and I respect the meaningful boundaries that allow a balanced life to flourish.
- I gain energy from my balanced approach to work, exercise, and time with family.

Behaviors That Support My Health

- I eat a clean, vegetarian diet.
- I sleep well.
- I read for pleasure and participate in recreational activities with my family.

STEP 3: SET 3-MONTH GOALS

Ask yourself the following questions:

- What is my current status in the area of my life that I want to focus on?

- What behaviors can I challenge myself to pursue consistently within 3 months to take me toward my vision?

Sample 3-Month Goals

- Related to the area of Fitness: I will be physically active for a total of 30 to 60 minutes, 3 to 5 days a week, including 3 days of only cardiovascular exercise and 2 days of both cardiovascular exercise and strength training.

- Related to the area of Life Balance: I will respect the boundaries of work, exercise, and leisure by finding two new ways to relax during my workday and one new way to have leisure time in my after-work hours; I will implement each of them one time per week.

- Related to the area of Behaviors That Support My Health: I will sleep an average of 7 to 8 hours per night, 5 to 6 days per week, by implementing strategies to improve both the amount and quality of my sleep.

STEPS 4 AND 5: SET WEEKLY GOALS AND MODIFY YOUR GOALS AS YOU GO

To begin, set the first weekly goals of your progression toward each of your 3-month goals. Assess your progress at the end of every week and set your goals for the following week. Make sure your goals are measurable and specific and that they help you move closer to meeting your 3-month goal.

3-Month Goal #1

I will be physically active for a total of 30 to 60 minutes, 3 to 5 days a week, including 3 days of only cardiovascular exercise and 2 days of both cardiovascular exercise and strength training.

Week 1 Goals

- I will research pedometers.
  Rationale: Positive step to ensure regular activity; putting number on activities throughout the day can be motivating.

- I will note the time it takes to walk around the lake near my house.
  Rationale: Establishes a baseline.

- I will purchase dumbbells and a stability ball for home use.
  Rationale: Positive step to ensure regular activity; makes exercise convenient (don't have to go to the gym).

Week 2 Goals

- I will wear the pedometer 2 or 3 days this week. (Refined goal: Researching pedometers is completed. Ready to raise the bar.)
  Rationale: Put the new pedometer to use.

- I will walk around the lake in under 45 minutes one or two times this week. (Refined goal: Measuring the time it takes to walk around the lake is completed. Ready to raise the bar.)
  Rationale: Found walk doable in 50 minutes. Challenge myself to walk faster.

- I will ride my bike for 40 to 60 minutes one time this week. (Added: Brand new cardio exercise goal.)
  Rationale: Wanted some variety in cardio workout.

- I will do a strength training workout three times this week, doing upper body exercises on Tuesday and Thursday and lower body exercises on Wednesday. (Refined goal: Purchasing dumbbells and a stability ball is completed. Ready to raise the bar.)
  Rationale: Put the new equipment to use.

Week 3 Goals

- I will wear the pedometer 2 or 3 days this week, aiming for at least 8,000 steps on each of those days. (Refined goal: Raises the bar of the goal of wearing a pedometer.)
  Rationale: Found baseline was an average of 7,500 steps per day. Included a steps-per-day goal to realistically increase that baseline.

- I will walk around the lake at a moderate pace one or two times this week. (Refined goal: Lowers the hurdle of walking around the lake in under 45 minutes.)

Rationale: Walking around the lake in 45 minutes felt like too much pressure. Felt exhausted afterward.

- I will ride my bike for 40 to 60 minutes one time this week. (Maintained goal: Kept the original goal the same.)
  Rationale: This goal is going well and feels very challenging.

- I will purchase a strength training DVD and train two or three times this week. (Eliminated goal: Dropped the goal of doing strength training on 3 days per week on my own, splitting my routine into upper and lower body workouts. Added goal: Brand new strength training goal.)
  Rationale: Need more visual assistance; believe that working my whole body at one time will work better.

3-Month Goal #2

I will respect the boundaries of work, exercise, and leisure by finding two new ways to relax during my workday and one new way to have leisure time in my after-work hours; I will implement each of them one time per week.

Week 1 Goals

- I will chart the average number of hours I spend in my office daily.
  Rationale: Establish a baseline. If I can "prove" that I can work less and still get my work done, it can help me stay motivated.

- I will eat lunch away from my office one or two times this week.
  Rationale: Begin to add variety to my habit of always eating at my desk.

- I will set an alarm to ring on my computer every 2 hours. When it rings, I will get up and move around, taking deep breaths and doing light stretches for 5 minutes.
  Rationale: Experiment to see if periodic movement helps me feel better and increases my energy.

Week 2 Goals

- I will chart the average number of hours I spend in my office daily. (Maintained goal: Kept the original goal the same.)

Rationale: Need to continue to track my hours to "prove" that I can work less and still get my work done.

- I will leave work by 5:30 p.m. 2 or 3 days this week. (Added goal: Brand new scheduling goal.)
  Rationale: A step toward having time for myself in the evenings.

- I will eat lunch away from my office 2 or 3 days this week. (Refined goal: Raises the bar on the goal to eat lunch away from my office one or two times per week.)
  Rationale: Like the variety this provides.

- I will set an alarm to ring on my computer every 2 hours. When it rings, I will get up and move around, taking deep breaths and doing light stretches for 5 minutes. (Maintained goal: Kept the original goal the same.)
  Rationale: Enjoyed this and felt great!

Week 3 Goals

- (Eliminated goal: Dropped the goal to chart the average number of hours I spend in my office daily.)
  Rationale: I can see that leaving at 5:30 p.m. on some days is going well. I am still getting my work done!

- I will eat lunch away from my office 3 or 4 days this week (Refined goal: Raises the bar on the goal to eat lunch away from my office 2 or 3 days per week.)
  Rationale: The change of environment has been good. I believe this will be one of my two ways to create time for myself during my workday.

- I will set an alarm to ring on my computer every 2 hours. When it rings, I will get up and move around, taking deep breaths and doing light stretches for 5 minutes. (Maintained goal: Kept the original goal the same.)
  Rationale: I believe this will be the second of my two ways to create time for myself during my workday.

- I will leave work by 5:30 p.m. on 2 or 3 days this week. (Maintained goal: Kept the original goal the same.)
  Rationale: I left early two times last week and my work productivity was still good.

3-Month Goal #3

I will sleep an average of 7 to 8 hours per night, 5 or 6 days per week, by implementing strategies to improve both the amount and quality of my sleep.

Week 1 Goals

- I will purchase a sleep journal.
  Rationale: A journal is necessary for me to accurately track my sleep patterns and the thoughts I'm having as I go to sleep.

- I will have a cup of calming tea before bed 4 to 6 nights this week.
  Rationale: Create a ritual to signal moving from daily routine to bedtime.

- I will meditate for 10 to 15 minutes before bedtime 5 days this week.
  Rationale: Meditating will help me relax before going to bed.

Week 2 Goals

- I will keep my sleep journal in the kitchen and write two to five sentences in it each morning while having coffee. (Refined goal: Purchasing sleep journal completed. Ready to raise the bar.)
  Rationale: Use the journal at a logical and convenient time.

- I will have a cup of calming tea and read a chapter of a book of my choosing before bed 4 to 6 nights this week. (Refined goal: Raises the bar of the original goal by adding an activity to the goal.)
  Rationale: Add another pleasurable activity to after-work time, further separating daily routine and bedtime.

- I will meditate on Monday, Wednesday, and Friday nights before bed using a guided meditation CD. (Refined goal: Lowered the bar of the goal to meditate 5 nights per week and added a supporting strategy to help increase likelihood of success.)
  Rationale: Meditation without guidance is challenging. Need structured practice.

Week 3 Goals

- I will keep my sleep journal in the kitchen and write two to five sentences each morning while having coffee. (Maintained goal: Kept the original goal the same.)

Rationale: Interesting practice that captures thoughts around sleep quantity and quality.

- I will have a cup of calming tea and read a chapter in a book of my choosing before bed 4 to 6 nights this week. (Maintained goal: Kept the goal the same.)
  Rationale: Bedtime routine seems to be helping improve my quality and quantity of sleep; also contributes to long-term wellness vision of reading for pleasure.

- I will do 10 to 20 minutes of restorative yoga (with a DVD) before bed on 1 to 3 nights this week. (Eliminated goal: Dropped goal of meditation on Monday, Wednesday, and Friday. Added goal: Brand new goal involving meditative practice.)
  Rationale: Meditation was not working. Yoga seems like a great combination of meditation and soothing physical activity.

- I will be in bed by 11:00 p.m. on 2 to 4 nights this week. (Added goal: Brand new scheduling goal.)
  Rationale: Noticed that 11:45 is average bedtime; need to get to bed earlier to increase quantity of sleep.

ACKNOWLEDGMENTS

We'd like to acknowledge our former colleagues at the Duke Diet & Fitness Center who taught us about the physical and emotional challenges involved with losing weight and, more important, how to support overweight individuals in the journey toward a healthier life. This book is a product of our time as a part of the incredible staff at Duke and we would like to acknowledge the role of each and every co-worker from that nascent period in our career, including Dr. Michael Hamilton, Franca Alphin, Peggy Norwood, Dr. Susan Head, and Dr. Ronnie Kolotkin.

Our deepest gratitude to Dr. Francesca Amati, who helped us present our ideas in at University Hospital in Geneva, Switzerland, nearly 10 years ago.

We'd like to thank our colleagues working on the Biggest Loser Club, Maria Patella and Louise Massey. Our synergy with these two wonderful ladies and incredible coaches helps us deliver a service to the BLC members that we can be very proud of. Big thanks to Joe Bilman for introducing us to the opportunities at Rodale and to David Krivda and Glenn Abel for helping us do what we love to do on the Biggest Loser Club. And much love to Melissa Roberson, the excellent editor of the Biggest Loser Club who has given us undying support as online experts.

To our colleagues in the field of wellness coaching, thanks for ongoing inspiration, including Margaret Moore, Julie Schwartz, Ellen Albertson, Frank Claps, Ellen Garrison, Mandy Hillstrom, Kati Konersman, Lynn Grieger, and Kevin Rail. Singular recognition to Blaine Wilson and Gloria Silverio, who went above and beyond in helping us edit the coaching section.

Also, thank you to our colleagues Louise Massey who reviewed the nutrition section and Monica Churchill and Charlene Reeves who reviewed the exercise guidelines. And special thanks to Amira Ranney and Greg Blais of Mountain Physical Therapy for their assistance with the fitness section.

A special thanks to our editors that helped shape our ideas into this book, starting with Julie Will for saying yes to our vision for *Coach Yourself Thin*, Jeff Kottiel for helping refine the proposal, Marianne McGinnis for helping us through the growing pains of the first draft, Tory Glerum and Erana Bumbardatore for doing the lion's share of the editing, and Marie Crousillat for guiding us in the final stages.

Our sincere appreciation to the following professionals for giving us permission to use their intellectual property: Dr. James Prochaska for his work with Dr. John Norcross and Dr. Carlo DiClemente, Dr. Jon Kabat-Zinn, Dr. Linda Craighead, Maria Patella, Dr. Susan Head, Lori Shepard, and Judy Wilson.

To our clients who shared their stories in *Coach Yourself Thin* and helped us bring the journey you are about to experience to life, we give our heartfelt thanks. And we are eternally grateful to the thousands of Biggest Loser Club members who put their trust in us over the past six years.

And finally, our hearts go out to our family and friends without whom the vision for this book would have never made it to print.

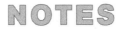

NOTES

Chapter 16

1. Kabat-Zinn, Jon. Full Catastrophe Living: Using the Wisdom of Your Body and Mind to Face Stress, Pain and Illness (New York: Delta, 1990), 27–29.

Chapter 18

1. Environmental Working Group, www.ewg.org/foodnews/summary.

Chapter 19

1. Linda W. Craighead, *The Appetite Awareness Workbook: How to Listen to Your Body and Overcome Bingeing, Overeating, and Obsession with Food* (Oakland, CA: New Harbinger, 2006).

Chapter 23

1. C. Tudor-Locke and D. R. Bassett Jr., "How many steps/day are enough? Preliminary pedometer indices for public health," *Sports Medicine* 34, no. 1 (2004): 1–8.

Chapter 24

1. J. E. Donnelly, et al, "American College of Sports Medicine position stand: Appropriate physical activity intervention strategies for weight loss and prevention of weight regain for adults," *Medicine and Science in Sports and Exercise* 41, vol 2 (2009): 459–71. Erratum in *Medicine and Science in Sports and Exercise* 41, no. 7: 1532.

2. *American College of Sports Medicine's Guidelines for Exercise Testing and Prescription,* 7th ed. (Philadelphia: Lippincott Williams & Wilkins, 2006).

3. Ibid.

4. Modified from Gunnar Borg, Borg's *Perceived Exertion and Pain Scales* (Champaign, IL: Human Kinetics, 1998).

Chapter 25

1. Guidelines adapted from Nicholas A. Ratamess, Ph.D, et al, "American College of Sports Medicine position stand: Progression models in resistance training for healthy adults," *Medicine and Science in Sports and Exercise* 41, vol. 3 (2009): 687–708

Chapter 27

1. J. O. Prochaska, J. C. Norcross, and C. C. DiClemente, *Changing for Good* (New York: Morrow, 1994).

Chapter 29

1. Adapted with permission from Dr. Susan Head, www.susanheadphd.com.

Chapter 31

1. Created by Maria Patella. Used with permission.

REFERENCES

American College of Sports Medicine. *ACSM's Guidelines for Exercise Testing and Prescription* (7th ed.). Philadelphia: Lippincott Williams & Wilkins, 2006.

American College of Sports Medicine. *ACSM Fitness Book* (3rd ed.). Human Kinetics, 2003

Bushman, Barbara A. *American College of Sports Medicine's Complete Guide to Fitness & Health.* Human Kinetics, 2011.

Craighead, Linda W. *The Appetite Awareness Workbook: How to Listen to Your Body and Overcome Bingeing, Overeating, and Obsession with Food* (Oakland, CA: New Harbinger, 2006).

Daly, A., and A. Evert. *Choose Your Foods: Exchange Lists for Weight Management.* The American Diabetes Association and the American Dietetic Association, 2007.

Donnelly, J. E., et al. "American College of Sports Medicine Position Stand: Appropriate Physical Activity Intervention Strategies for Weight Loss and Prevention of Weight Regain for Adults," Medicine and Science in Sports and Exercise 41, no. 2 (Feb. 2009).

Kabat-Zinn, Jon. *Full Catastrophe Living: Using the Wisdom of Your Body and Mind to Face Stress, Pain and Illness.* New York: Delta, 1990.

Kravitz, Len. "The 25 Most Significant Health Benefits of Physical Activity & Exercise." *IDEA Fitness Journal* 4, no. 9 (October 2007).

Louv, Richard. *The Nature Principle: Human Restoration and the End of Nature-Deficit Disorder.* New York: Algonquin Books of Chapel Hill, Workman Publishing, 2011.

Orem, S., J. Binkert, and A. Clancy. *Appreciative Coaching: A Positive Process for Change.* San Francisco: Jossey-Bass, 2007.

Prochaska, J. O., J. C. Norcross, , and C. C. DiClemente. *Changing for Good.* New York: Morrow, 1994.

Whitney, D., and A. Trosten-Bloom. *The Power of Appreciative Inquiry: A Practical Guide to Positive Change.* San Francisco: Berrett-Koehler, 2003.

RESOURCES

GENERAL

Head, S., and S. Nilsen. *Winning at Weight Loss: How to Achieve Lifelong Weight-Management and Physical Fitness*, 2004. Available through www.susanheadphd.com.

The American College of Sports Medicine (ACSM) and the American Heart Association (AHA) Physical Activity and Public Health Guidelines.

The 2008 Physical Activity Guidelines for Americans.

Evaluate your personal strengths: www.authentichappiness.sas.upenn.edu/Default.aspx

Examples of exercises:

www.acefitness.org/exerciselibrary/default.aspx

www.livestrong.com/ (*Note:* Enter "How to do" plus the name of the exercise—squat, bench press, lunge, lat pulldown, etc.—in the search tool.)

www.ideafit.com/exercise-library

Healthy Heart Information: www.heart.org/HEARTORG/

Heart rate monitors: www.polarusa.com

National Diabetes Information Clearinghouse: diabetes.niddk.nih.gov/

Pedometers: www.accusplit.com

Vegetarian Resource Group: www.vrg.org

EMOTIONAL EATING BOOKS

Albers, S. *50 Ways to Soothe Yourself without Food.* Oakland, CA: New Harbinger, 2009.

Craighead, Linda W. *The Appetite Awareness Workbook: How to Listen to Your Body and Overcome Bingeing, Overeating, and Obsession with Food.* Oakland, CA: New Harbinger, 2006.

Loring, Sasha T. *Eating with Fierce Kindness: A Mindful and Compassionate Guide to Losing Weight.* Oakland, CA: New Harbinger, 2010.

EMOTIONAL EATING TREATMENT CENTERS

Renfrew Center: www.renfrewcenter.com/

River Oaks Hospital Eating Disorders Treatment Center: www.riveroakshospital.com

FIND A PROFESSIONAL

Coach Yourself Thin classes: www.novowellness.com

Cognitive behavior therapist: www.nacbt.org/searchfortherapists.asp

Dietitian: www.eatright.org/programs/rdfinder/

Personal trainer:

http://forms.acsm.org/__frm/crt/online__locator.asp

www.acefitness.org/findanacepro/default.aspx

Wellness coach: www.wellcoaches.com/

INDEX